Lipids

Editor

DONALD A. SMITH

ENDOCRINOLOGY AND METABOLISM CLINICS OF NORTH AMERICA

www.endo.theclinics.com

Consulting Editor
DEREK LeROITH

December 2014 • Volume 43 • Number 4

ELSEVIER

1600 John F. Kennedy Boulevard • Suite 1800 • Philadelphia, Pennsylvania, 19103-2899

http://www.theclinics.com

ENDOCRINOLOGY AND METABOLISM CLINICS OF NORTH AMERICA Volume 43, Number 4
December 2014 ISSN 0889-8529, ISBN 13: 978-0-323-32646-9

Editor: Jessica McCool
Developmental Editor: Susan Showalter

Endocrinology and Metabolism Clinics of North America (ISSN 0889-8529) is published quarterly by Elsevier Inc., 360 Park Avenue South, New York, NY 10010-1710. Months of issue are March, June, September, and December. Periodicals postage paid at New York, NY and additional mailing offices. Subscription prices are USD 330.00 per year for US individuals, USD 581.00 per year for US institutions, USD 165.00 per year for US students and residents, USD 415.00 per year for Canadian individuals, USD 718.00 per year for Canadian institutions, USD 480.00 per year for international individuals, USD 718.00 per year for international institutions, and USD 245.00 per year for international and Canadian and foreign students/residents. To receive student/resident rate, orders must be accompanied by name of affiliated institution, date of term, and the signature of program/residency coordinator on institution letterhead. Orders will be billed at individual rate until proof of status is received. Foreign air speed delivery is included in all *Clinics* subscription prices. All prices are subject to change without notice. **POSTMASTER:** Send address changes to *Endocrinology and Metabolism Clinics of North America*, Elsevier Health Sciences Division, Subscription Customer Service, 3251 Riverport Lane, Maryland Heights, MO 63043. **Customer Service: Telephone: 1-800-654-2452** (U.S. and Canada); **1-314-447-8871** (outside U.S. and Canada). **Fax: 1-314-447-8029. E-mail: journalscustomerservice-usa@elsevier.com** (for print support); **journalsonlinesupport-usa@elsevier.com** (for online support).

Reprints. For copies of 100 or more, of articles in this publication, please contact the Commercial Rights Department, Elsevier Inc., 360 Park Avenue South, New York, NY 10010-1710; phone: +1-212-633-3874; fax: +1-212-633-3820; E-mail: reprints@elsevier.com.

Endocrinology and Metabolism Clinics of North America is covered in *MEDLINE/PubMed (Index Medicus)*, *EMBASE/Excerpta Medica*, *Current Contents/Clinical Medicine*, *Current Contents/Life Sciences*, *Science Citation Index*, *ISI/BIOMED*, *BIOSIS*, and *Chemical Abstracts*.

Contributors

CONSULTING EDITOR

DEREK LeROITH, MD, PhD
Director of Research, Division of Endocrinology, Metabolism, and Bone Diseases, Department of Medicine, Icahn School of Medicine at Mount Sinai, New York, New York

EDITOR

DONALD A. SMITH, MD, MPH, FACP, FNLA, FACE
Associate Professor of Medicine and Preventive Medicine, Icahn School of Medicine at Mount Sinai, New York, New York

AUTHORS

JUAN J. BADIMON, PhD
Cardiovascular Institute, Icahn School of Medicine at Mount Sinai, New York, New York

MICHAEL B. BOFFA, PhD
Associate Professor, Department of Chemistry and Biochemistry, University of Windsor, Windsor, Ontario, Canada

MICHAEL DAVIDSON, MD
Section of Cardiology, University of Chicago, Chicago, Illinois

ARPETA GUPTA, MD
Fellow, Division of Endocrinology, Diabetes, and Bone Diseases, Icahn School of Medicine at Mount Sinai, New York, New York

HARVEY S. HECHT, MD, FACC, FSCCT
Associate Director of Cardiovascular Imaging, Department of Cardiology, Mount Sinai Medical Center; Professor of Medicine, Icahn School of Medicine at Mount Sinai, New York, New York

PHILIP K. JOHNSON, BS
Department of Cardiology, Boston Children's Hospital; Department of Pediatrics, Harvard Medical School, Boston, Massachusetts

MARLYS L. KOSCHINSKY, PhD
Dean, Faculty of Science; and Professor, Department of Chemistry and Biochemistry, University of Windsor, Windsor, Ontario, Canada

PENNY M. KRIS-ETHERTON, PhD, RD
Distinguished Professor of Nutrition, Department of Nutritional Sciences, The Pennsylvania State University, University Park, Pennsylvania

FREDERICK J. RAAL, MBBCh, MMED, PhD
Department of Medicine, Faculty of Health Sciences, University of the Witwatersrand, Johannesburg, South Africa

CHESNEY K. RICHTER, BS, PhD(c)
Department of Nutritional Sciences, The Pennsylvania State University, University Park, Pennsylvania

ROBERT S. ROSENSON, MD
Cardiovascular Institute, Icahn School of Medicine at Mount Sinai, New York, New York

CARLOS G. SANTOS-GALLEGO, MD
Cardiovascular Institute, Icahn School of Medicine at Mount Sinai, New York, New York

AMITA SINGH, MD
Section of Cardiology, University of Chicago, Chicago, Illinois

ANN C. SKULAS-RAY, PhD
Research Associate, Department of Nutritional Sciences, The Pennsylvania State University, University Park, Pennsylvania

DONALD A. SMITH, MD, MPH, FACP, FNLA, FACE
Associate Professor of Medicine and Preventive Medicine, Icahn School of Medicine at Mount Sinai, New York, New York

EVAN A. STEIN, MD, PhD
Metabolic and Atherosclerosis Research Center, Cincinnati, Ohio

JUSTIN P. ZACHARIAH, MD, MPH
Department of Cardiology, Boston Children's Hospital; Department of Pediatrics, Harvard Medical School, Boston, Massachusetts

Contents

The 2013 American College of Cardiology/American Heart Association
Guideline on the Treatment of Blood Cholesterol to Reduce Atherosclerotic Cardiovascular Risk in Adults and Guideline on the Assessment of
Cardiovascular Risk were released in mid-November 2013. This article
explains the guidelines, the risk equations, and their derivations, and addresses criticisms so that practicing physicians may be more comfortable
in using the guidelines and the risk equations to inform patients of their
atherosclerotic cardiovascular risk and choices to reduce that risk. The
article also addresses patient concerns about statin safety if lifestyle
changes have been insufficient to reduce their risk.

Coronary artery calcium scanning (CAC) is the most powerful prognosti-
cator of cardiac risk in the asymptomatic primary prevention population,
far exceeding the role of risk factor–based paradigms. The primary utility
of risk factors is to identify treatable targets for risk reduction after risk
has been determined by CAC. Serial calcium scanning to evaluate progression of calcified plaque is useful for determining the response to treatment. The 2013 cholesterol treatment guidelines understate the value of
CAC scanning for atherosclerotic disease risk assessment.

This article reconciles the classic view of high-density lipoproteins (HDL)
associated with low risk for cardiovascular disease (CVD) with recent
data (genetics studies and randomized clinical trials) casting doubt over
the widely accepted beneficial role of HDL regarding CVD risk. Although
HDL cholesterol has been used as a surrogate measure to investigate
HDL function, the cholesterol content in HDL particles is not an indicator
of the atheroprotective properties of HDL. Thus, more precise measures
of HDL metabolism are needed to reflect and account for the beneficial

effects of HDL particles. Current and emerging therapies targeting HDL are discussed.

Marlys L. Koschinsky and Michael B. Boffa

Elevated plasma concentrations of lipoprotein(a) (Lp[a]) are an emerging risk factor for the development of coronary heart disease (CHD). Recent genetic and epidemiologic data have provided strong evidence for a causal role of Lp(a) in CHD. Despite these developments, which have attracted increasing interest from clinicians and basic scientists, many unanswered questions persist. The true pathogenic mechanism of Lp(a) remains a mystery. Significant uncertainty exists concerning the appropriate use of Lp(a) in the clinical setting. No therapeutic intervention exists that can specifically lower plasma Lp(a) concentrations, although the list of compounds that lower Lp(a) and LDL continues to expand.

Chesney K. Richter, Ann C. Skulas-Ray, and Penny M. Kris-Etherton

There is extensive evidence from epidemiologic studies and clinical trials demonstrating that the Mediterranean dietary pattern reduces the risk of many chronic diseases, including cardiovascular disease (CVD), and the attendant risk factors. A Mediterranean-style diet reflects most food and nutrient goals in current dietary guidelines. Minor modifications to reduce sodium and saturated fat intake can be made to further meet recommendations. Including the Mediterranean diet in the list of recommended evidence-based dietary patterns offers an additional strategy for improving dietary habits, which may help individuals achieve better long-term adherence to dietary guidelines and sustain optimal reductions in CVD risk.

Justin P. Zachariah and Philip K. Johnson

The National Heart, Lung and Blood Institute Expert Panel Integrated Guidelines promote the prevention of cardiovascular disease (CVD) events by encouraging healthy behaviors in all children, screening and treatment of children with genetic dyslipidemias, usage of specific lifestyle modifications, and limited administration of lipid pharmacotherapy in children with the highest CVD risk. These recommendations place children in the center of the fight against future CVD. Pediatric providers may be in a position to shift the focus of CVD prevention from trimming multiple risk factors to attacking the roots of CVD.

Amita Singh and Michael Davidson

Many lipid-lowering drugs improve cardiovascular (CV) outcomes. However, when therapies have been studied in addition to statins, it has been challenging to show an additional clinical benefit in terms of CV event reduction, although overall safety seems acceptable. This debate has been complicated by recent guidelines that emphasize treatment with high-potency statin monotherapy. Combination therapy allows more patients to successfully reach their ideal lipid targets. Further testing of novel therapies may introduce an era of potent low-density lipoprotein decrease without dependence on statins, but until then, they remain the mainstay of therapy.

Although the past 4 decades have been the most productive in transitioning from an low-density lipoprotein cholesterol (LDL-C) hypothesis to demonstration of clinical benefit, cardiovascular disease remains a major cause of mortality and morbidity. It is fortunate that most of the effective lipid-lowering drugs, the statins, have become generic and inexpensive. However, there remains a large unmet medical need for new and effective agents that are also well tolerated and safe, especially for patients unable to either tolerate statins or achieve optimal LDL-C on current therapies. It is likely that the agents discussed in this review will fill that need.

ENDOCRINOLOGY AND METABOLISM CLINICS OF NORTH AMERICA

RELATED INTEREST

Cardiology Clinics, Volume 32, Issue 3 (August 2014)
Coronary Artery Disease
David M. Shavelle, *Editor*
Available at: http://www.cardiology.theclinics.com/

VISIT THE CLINICS ONLINE!
Access your subscription at:
www.theclinics.com

Foreword

Lipids 2014: New Guidelines, New Concepts, New Diets, New Drugs

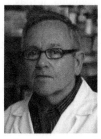

Derek LeRoith, MD, PhD
Consulting Editor

Dr Smith has compiled a lipids issue that is extremely timely for the practicing endocrinologist as the field of clinical lipidology is rapidly evolving with new guidelines by AHA/ACC, new concepts in risk assessment, HDL and Lp(a), new dietary plans, unexpected large outcome trial results, and new medications in the pipeline. The topics that were chosen reflect these issues.

Drs Gupta and Smith open the issue with an article aimed at simplifying the new ACC/AHA guidelines that were released in November 2013. The important question facing the primary care physician is whom should be treated with statin therapy, in addition to lifestyle modifications, and how intensively. Individuals with diabetes or very high LDL levels and those with atherosclerotic cardiovascular disease (ASCVD) should receive moderate to intensive therapy to prevent primary or secondary ASCVD. In 2013, the ACC/AHA developed race- and sex-specific 10-year risk equations as well as lifetime equations for ASCVD to help primary-prevention decision-making by health care professionals and their patients. These guidelines replace the earlier Framingham risk equations for coronary heart disease based on a largely white population.

Coronary artery calcium score has proven to be extremely useful in the primary prevention of coronary artery disease. Evidence presented by Dr Hecht actually suggests it may be more valuable than relying on classic risk factor assessment. Furthermore, the radiation exposure from this CT-related technique has been lowered to that no greater than a screening mammogram. As discussed in his article, while reimbursement for the procedure is not readily available, the cost is low, and it often reclassifies ASCVD risk assessed by standard risk factor–based paradigms and thus should be used more widely.

Traditionally, HDL-cholesterol was considered protective against cardiovascular disease (CVD). However, this assumption has been partially disproved by recent

Endocrinol Metab Clin N Am 43 (2014) ix–xi
http://dx.doi.org/10.1016/j.ecl.2014.09.002
0889-8529/14/$ – see front matter

evidence and replaced by the suggestion that HDL-cholesterol levels do not actually measure HDL functionality. It would therefore be more appropriate to measure HDL particles, as describe in the article by Drs Santos-Gallego, Badimon, and Rosenson. This measurement gives a more functional estimate and may partly explain the failure of certain trials that increase HDL-C levels (eg, combining niacin with statins) to prevent CVD. More recent attempts to increase HDL particles (eg, with CETP blockers) may be more effective in CVD prevention.

Drs Kochinsky and Boffa describe the recent interest in lipoprotein(a) as a risk factor for CVD. While it may not be appropriate for screening large populations, it may be valuable in the management of the individual patients. Lp(a) may also be partially cleared by the LDL receptor and therefore affected by statin therapy and an emerging therapy being tested, namely, the PCSK9 inhibitors. The mechanism whereby Lp(a) may affect CVD is still being explored and clinical trials on its specific inhibition can only be carried out once specific inhibitors are available.

Recent studies have suggested that the classic Mediterranean diet with increased olive oil or nuts can achieve long-term dietary adherence and reduce ASCVD outcomes compared with the classic American low-fat diet. As discussed by Drs Richter, Skulas-Ray, and Kris-Etherton, the Mediterranean diet closely correlates with dietary guidelines recommended by the new AHA/ACC guidelines for prevention of CVD, with the only extra requirements being the attention to salt intake and fat composition of the diets.

Drs Zachariah and Johnson discuss the importance of considering monitoring and treating dyslipidemia in the pediatric age group. There are a number of causes for the dyslipidemia, some genetic, some secondary to diseases or medications, but no less important are the dyslipidemias associated with lifestyle factors. Despite the concern that monitoring dyslipidemia may lead to unnecessary medications, one factor to be considered is that dyslipidemia in childhood may in fact be a cause of atherosclerosis in early adulthood. Thus, the recommendations are to measure lipids, intensify lifestyle changes as much as possible, and consider medications where indicated.

Drs Singh and Davidson discuss the issue of combination therapies in the management of dyslipidemia. The AHA/ACC 2013 guidelines do not specifically discuss this area except to state that combination therapy is available when goals are not met using statin therapies or there are statin-related adverse events. Niacin, fibrates, ezetimibe, and fish oils have been or are being tested in combination with statin therapy for ASCVD prevention. While most are apparently safe and have effects on various lipid parameters, their added efficacy over the statin use alone has come into question. PSCK9 inhibitors show great promise and are being tested in ASCVD event trials in combination with statin therapy.

Statin therapy has been, and remains, the mainstay of therapy to reduce the levels of LDL-cholesterol and thereby significantly reduce CVD. Since most statins are now generic and therefore available to most individuals, their use worldwide has led to remarkable preventive results. As described by Drs Stein and Raal, there are rare patients with Homozygous Familial Hypercholesterolemia who have such abnormal LDL receptors that statins are relatively ineffective in lowering LDL-cholesterol. Newer agents such as mipomersen and lomitapide decrease hepatic VLDL and subsequent LDLC synthesis and now have limited FDA approval for use in such patients. There are other patients that are statin-averse, either due to intolerable side effects such as myalgias or more recently fear of inducing diabetes. Alternatives are available but are much less effective, and thus, other agents are being developed as alternatives or to be used in combination with statins for greater efficacy. The most exciting new classes of agents include the PSCK9 inhibitors and the CETP inhibitors. PSCK9 inhibition results in increased hepatic LDL receptor expression and significant LDL-cholesterol lowering. The CETP inhibitors increase HDL-cholesterol and decrease LDL-cholesterol in varying degrees. Event trials are proceeding in both classes.

Dr Smith and the authors of each article should be applauded for their outstanding contributions, bringing to the reader the latest issues confronting us in the field of lipidology and presenting the information and clinical applicability so clearly.

Derek LeRoith, MD, PhD
Division of Endocrinology, Metabolism, and Bone Diseases
Department of Medicine
Icahn School of Medicine at Mount Sinai
One Gustave L. Levy Place
Box 1055, Altran 4-36
New York, NY 10029, USA

E-mail address:
derek.leroith@mssm.edu

Preface

Lipids

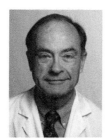

Donald A. Smith, MD, MPH, FACP, FNLA, FACE
Editor

After almost 50 years of lipid-altering clinical trials with numerous drugs and diets, one would think that the practice of clinical lipidology had stabilized. But, as in all medicine, just when treatments and goals seem certain and accepted, they change.

Such has been the case with lipids in the last 5 years:

1. Dietary trials suggest a more Mediterranean, less lipid-stingy, dietary preventive approach.
2. A newer view of screening and managing lipids in children has been adopted and promoted.
3. New 10-year and lifetime predictive equations for myocardial infarction, coronary death, and stroke have been derived from 5 cohort studies more racially inclusive than the Framingham Study to assist physicians and patients determine the need for statin preventive therapy.
4. Clinical trial statin data have focused the new AHA/ACC guidelines on high- and medium-dose statin therapy rather than determining dosing based on lipid goals.
5. Coronary calcium score imaging's lower cost and radiation dosing have now enabled its use to sharpen coronary risk prediction.
6. The roles of the increasingly complex lipoproteins, HDL and Lp(a), in atherosclerosis continue to be explored.
7. Recent clinical add-on trials of niacin and fibric acid to statins have been disappointing, but
8. Recent clinical trials of
   a. New orphan lipid-altering medications, a microsomal triglyceride transfer protein inhibitor and an Apo-B antisense oligonucleotide, and
   b. Proprotein convertase subtilisin/kexin type 9 inhibitors have been extremely exciting and may satisfy the needs of patients for whom statins are insufficient or problematic.

Endocrinol Metab Clin N Am 43 (2014) xiii–xiv
http://dx.doi.org/10.1016/j.ecl.2014.09.001
0889-8529/14/$ – see front matter © 2014 Published by Elsevier Inc.

endo.theclinics.com

It is these issues—new guidelines, new concepts, new diets, new drugs—about which I have asked the contributors to write for the interested endocrinologist and clinical practitioner to keep abreast of a rapidly changing field. I trust you will find them helpful.

Donald A. Smith, MD, MPH, FACP, FNLA, FACE
Associate Professor of Medicine and Preventive Medicine
Icahn School of Medicine at Mount Sinai
1 Gustave Levy Place, Box 1014
New York, NY 10029-6574, USA

E-mail address:
donald.smith@mssm.edu

The 2013 American College of Cardiology/American Heart Association Guidelines on Treating Blood Cholesterol and Assessing Cardiovascular Risk

A Busy Practitioner's Guide

CrossMark

Arpeta Gupta, MD[a], Donald A. Smith, MD, MPH[b],*

KEYWORDS

- 2013 ACC/AHA cholesterol guidelines • Pooled cohort equations
- Ten-year ASCVD risk • Statin therapy • Primary prevention of ASCVD
- Blood cholesterol guideline • Cardiovascular risk guideline

KEY POINTS

- The 2013 American College of Cardiology/American Heart Association practice guidelines on the treatment of blood cholesterol and assessment of risk now include stroke in addition to coronary heart disease.
- New risk assessment equations for both 10-year and lifetime risk for atherosclerotic cardiovascular disease (ASCVD) events that include African Americans have been developed.
- Moderate-dose to high-dose statins are recommended for specific groups of persons; those greater than or equal to 21 years of age and low-density lipoprotein cholesterol greater than or equal to 190 mg/dL, and those 40 to 75 years of age with clinical ASCVD, diabetes, or 10-year ASCVD risk greater than or equal to 7.5%.
- New lifetime ASCVD risk equations may be useful in individuals 20 to 59 years of age and with less than 7.5% 10-year risk.
- Intensity of statin therapy can be modified based on probability of adverse statin side effects.

Disclosure: None (A. Gupta); Site Principal Investigator, Sanofi-Regeneron Odyssey trial (PCSK9 Inhibitor) (D.A. Smith).
[a] Division of Endocrinology, Diabetes, and Bone Diseases, Icahn School of Medicine at Mount Sinai, Box 1055, New York, NY 10029, USA; [b] Mount Sinai Heart, Icahn School of Medicine, Box 1014, 1 Gustave Levy Place, New York, NY 10029-6574, USA
* Corresponding author.
E-mail address: donald.smith@mssm.edu

Endocrinol Metab Clin N Am 43 (2014) 869–892
http://dx.doi.org/10.1016/j.ecl.2014.08.006
0889-8529/14/$ – see front matter © 2014 Elsevier Inc. All rights reserved.

Cardiovascular disease (CVD) remains the leading cause of morbidity and mortality, accounting for every 1 in 3 deaths in the United States.[1] Over the last decade, death rates attributable to CVD declined 31.0% and the number of CVD deaths per year declined by 16.7%. Death rates in 2010 attributable to stroke and coronary heart disease (CHD) were 39.1 and 113.6 down from 60.9 (−33%) and 186.8 (−36%) per 100,000 in 2000, respectively. In diabetic patients from 1990 to 2010 acute myocardial changes decreased 67.8%, stroke 52.7%, and amputations 51.4%.[2] However, in 2010, CVD still accounted for 31.9% of all deaths in the United States. A recent report from a national American clinical laboratory (Quest) reported on low-density lipoprotein (LDL) cholesterol (LDL-C) levels in 150 million Americans from 2000 to 2011. Although there was a steady decline from 2000 to 2008, LDL-C levels remained the same from 2008 to 2011, with no change in the percentage achieving any LDL-C goal levels, including levels less than 100 mg/dL.[3]

On 13 November, 2013, the Joint Task Force of the American College of Cardiology (ACC) and the American Heart Association (AHA) published new atherosclerotic CVD (ASCVD) prevention guidelines as an update to the 2008 guidelines developed by the National Heart, Lung, and Blood Institute.[4] This article restates the guidelines in a simpler format than the original synopsis[5] and discusses further the new risk equations that can help physicians and patients make decisions on lifestyle and medications to significantly reduce patients' lifetime risks of ASCVD.

PARADIGM SHIFT FROM TREAT-TO-TARGET TO INTENSITY OF STATIN THERAPY

For more than a decade, physicians have targeted LDL-C and non–high-density lipoprotein (HDL) cholesterol (non–HDL-C) goals by frequent laboratory testing, adjusting intensity of statin therapy, and using therapeutically unproven combinations of lipid-altering medication added to statin therapy. Unlike Adult Treatment Panel III (ATP-III) guidelines and the recent European and Canadian guidelines, the updated guidelines abandon these targets and recommend treating cholesterol by prescribing the appropriate intensity of statin therapy for those patients who are most likely to benefit. The panel's decision for this recommendation is based on a rigorous systematic review of randomized controlled trials (RCTs), a few of which are listed in **Table 1**; systematic reviews; and meta-analyses (**Table 2**) rather than fewer RCTs and expert opinion, which were used by the ATP-III guidelines. The recommendation is to measure LDL-C at baseline and rule out severe hypertriglyceridemia (≥500 mg/dL), reassess LDL-C 1 to 3 months after statin initiation and every 3 to 12 months thereafter to check for compliance (ie, the stability of the expected percentage decreases in LDL-C). Routine monitoring of alanine aminotransferase (ALT) or creatine phosphokinase (CPK) is no longer recommended in asymptomatic patients. This recommendation translates into less frequent laboratory testing, fewer dose adjustments, and less use of combination lipid therapy.

Previous calculators have defined clinical ASCVD as acute coronary syndromes, myocardial infarction (MI), stable angina, coronary or other arterial revascularization, stroke, transient ischemic attack (TIA), or peripheral arterial disease presumed to be of atherosclerotic origin. The current calculator focuses on so-called hard ASCVD, including first occurrence of nonfatal MI, death from CHD, and nonfatal and fatal stroke.

High-intensity statin therapy is defined as that producing greater than or equal to 50% reduction in LDL-C, with moderate-intensity statin therapy producing 30% to less than 50% reduction. Therefore, high-intensity statin therapy is recommended for groups of patients who are most likely to experience the greatest margin of benefit from the reduction in ASCVD risk given the greater potential for adverse effects.

Moderate-intensity statin therapy is recommended when conditions influencing safety are present (eg, in those >75 years of age), or in primary prevention patients less likely to experience a net benefit from high-intensity statin therapy.

If a less-than-anticipated reduction in LDL-C occurs after initiating a statin, lifestyle and drug adherence should be readdressed. Statin therapy may be uptitrated as tolerated. The addition of nonstatin therapy may also be considered in selected individuals.

Four groups of patients have been identified for whom strong evidence supports the use of statin therapy:

1. Clinical ASCVD
    i. Age less than or equal to 75 years and no safety concerns: high-intensity statin
    ii. Age greater than 75 years or less than or equal to 75 years with safety concerns: moderate-intensity statin
2. Primary prevention: primary LDL-C greater than or equal to 190 mg/dL
    i. Age greater than or equal to 21 years: high-intensity statin
3. Primary prevention: diabetes, age 40–75 years and LDL-C 70–189 mg/dL
    i. Moderate-intensity statin
    ii. Consider high-intensity statin when greater than or equal to 7.5% 10-year ASCVD risk using the pooled cohort equations
4. Primary prevention: no diabetes, age 40–75 years, LDL-C 70–189 mg/dL
    Always engage in a discussion about the risks and benefits of starting statin therapy.
    i. Greater than or equal to 7.5% 10-year ASCVD risk: moderate-intensity or high-intensity statin
    ii. Ten-year ASCVD risk, 5% to less than 7.5%: moderate-intensity statin
    iii. Individuals with less than 5% 10-year ASCVD risk may consider other factors:
        a. LDL-C greater than or equal to 160 mg/dL
        b. Evidence of genetic hyperlipidemias
        c. Family history of premature ASCVD with onset before 55 years of age in a first-degree male relative or before 65 years of age in a first-degree female relative
        d. High-sensitivity C-reactive protein (hs-CRP) greater than or equal to 2 mg/L
        e. Coronary artery calcium (CAC) score greater than or equal to 300 Agatston units or greater than or equal to 75th percentile for age, sex, and ethnicity
        f. Ankle-brachial index (ABI) less than 0.9
        g. High lifetime risk of ASCVD

In summary, all individuals with known CVD qualify to receive statins. For primary prevention, all individuals aged 21 years or older with an LDL-C level of 190 mg/dL or more qualify to receive statin therapy. Otherwise, clinicians should wait until patients are aged 40 years and start statins in those with LDL-C levels as low as 70 mg/dL if they have diabetes or have a calculated 10-year risk score for CVD of 7.5% or higher. For those suspected of having a higher risk than that calculated by the 10-year pooled cohort risk equation, other historical, biochemical, imaging, or risk equation factors listed earlier may be used.

Two groups of patients have not been shown to experience an ASCVD event reduction benefit from the routine initiation of statin therapy: those with New York Heart Association Class II to IV heart failure and those undergoing maintenance hemodialysis.

INCREASE IN ELIGIBILITY FOR STATIN THERAPY

Pencina and colleagues[6] analyzed 3773 National Health and Nutrition Examination Survey (NHANES) participants from 2005 to 2010 for statin eligibility based on the

Table 1
Some important statin trials for LDL-C goal setting

Trial	N	M/F (%)	Mean Age (y)	Medications	Primary vs Secondary Prevention	F/U (y)	Baseline Mean LDL-C mM/L	mg/dL	Achieved LDL-C in Statin Arm mM/L	mg/dL	Events	Relative Risk (CI)
Scandinavian Simvastatin Survival Study[40]	4444	82/18	58	Simvastatin 20/40 vs PBO	Secondary	5.0	4.9	196	3.2	127	All deaths All coronary deaths MI, CHD death Coronary revascularization	0.70 (0.58–0.85) 0.58 (0.46–0.73) 0.73 (0.66–0.80) 0.63 (0.54–0.74)
Heart Protection Study[41]	20,536	72/25	40–80	Simvastatin 40 vs PBO	Primary (DM ± hypertension) and secondary	5.4	3.4	136	2.4	96	Vascular deaths MI, CHD death Any stroke	0.83 (0.75–0.91) 0.73 (0.67–0.79) 0.75 (0.66–0.85)
Treating to New Targets[42]	10,001	81/19	35–75	Atorvastatin 80 vs 10	Secondary	4.9	2.6	101	2.0	77	MI, CHD death Any stroke	0.78 (0.68–0.91) 0.75 (0.59–0.96)
Anglo-Scandinavian Cholesterol Outcomes Trial, Lipid-lowering Arm[43]	10,305 hypertension + 3 additional RFs	81/19	40–79	Atorvastatin 10 vs PBO	Primary (15% previous stroke or PAD)	3.3	3.4	132	2.3	90	MI, CHD death Any stroke	0.64 (0.50–0.83) 0.73 (0.56–0.96)

Study	Population	M/F	Age	Drug	Prevention						Endpoint	HR (CI)
Collaborative Atorvastatin Diabetes Study[44]	2838 type 2 DM + 1 additional RF + LDL-C ≤160 + LDL-C ≤100	68/32	40–75	Atorvastatin 10 vs PBO	Primary	3.9	3.1	120	2.1	81	Acute CHD, coronary revascularization, stroke	0.63 (0.48–0.83)
											—	0.74 ($P<.05$)
Justification for the Use of Statins in Prevention: An Intervention Trial Evaluating Rosuvastatin[45]	17,902 LDL-C <130 hs-CRP ≥2.0	62/38	M>50 F>60	Rosuvastatin 20 vs PBO	Primary	1.9	2.8	110	1.4	55	MI, CVA, CV death, hospitalization for angina, revascularization	0.56 (0.46–0.69)
											All-cause mortality	0.80 (0.67–0.97)

Abbreviations: CI, confidence interval; CVA, cerebrovascular accident; DM, diabetes mellitus; F, female; F/U, follow-up; hs-CRP, high-sensitivity C-reactive protein; M, male; MI, myocardial infarction; PAD, peripheral artery disease; PBO, placebo; RF, risk factor.

Data from Refs.[40–45]

Table 2
Meta-analysis: efficacy and safety of intensive lowering of LDL-C from 170,000 participants in 26 randomized trials after ischemic vascular events

Study Design	Trial (n)	Subjects (n) Primary	Secondary	Baseline Mean LDL-C mM/L	mg/dL	LDL-C at 1 y in Statin Arm mM/L	mg/dL	F/U (y)	Vascular Events (% per Annum) PBO	Statin	Relative Risk Reduction % (CI)	Weighted RRR % per 40 mg/dL (1 mM/L) Lowering LDL-C (CI)
Total Vascular Events												
Combined	26	169,138										22 (20–24)
More vs less intensive	5	30,593	8659	2.6	101	2.1	81	5.1	5.3	4.5	15 (11–18)	28 (22–34)
Statin vs control	21	129,526		3.8	148	2.7	105	4.8	3.6	2.8	22 (19–24)	21 (19–23)
Any Major Coronary Event (Nonfatal MI, CHD Death)												
More vs less intensive	5	—		—		—		—	—		13 (7–19)	26 (15–35)
Statin vs control	21	—		—		—		—	—		27 (23–30)	24 (21–27)
Any Stroke												
More vs less intensive	5	—		—		—		—	—		1.4 (4–23)	26 (8–41)
Statin vs control	21	—		—		—		—	—		1.5 (9–20)	15 (10–20)
Revascularization (CABG, PTCA, Unspecified)												
More vs less intensive	5	—		—		—		—	—		19 (15–24)	34 (23–40)
Statin vs control	21	—		—		—		—	—		25 (21–28)	24 (20–27)

Abbreviations: CABG, coronary artery bypass grafting; PTCA, percutaneous transluminal coronary angioplasty.
Data from Cholesterol Treatment Trialists' (CTT) Collaboration, Baigent C, Blackwell L, Emberson J, et al. Efficacy and safety of more intensive lowering of LDL cholesterol: a meta-analysis of data from 170,000 participants in 26 randomised trials. Lancet 2010;376(9753):1670–81. http://dx.doi.org/10.1016/S0140-6736(10)61350-5.

new guidelines and extrapolated their results to 115.4 million US adults between the ages of 40 and 75 years. According to their calculations, 13 million more people would potentially be started on cholesterol-lowering medication under the new guidelines. Reasons for this increase include the reduction of the 10-year risk threshold from 10% to 7.5%, including stroke in the risk equations, and decreasing LDL-C treatment initiation threshold to 70 mg/dL. The investigators also note that most of this increase is in the older population where 87.4% of men and 53.6% of women between the ages of 60 and 75 years are now eligible to receive statin therapy. These numbers are an increase of 33% in men and 21.2% in women in this age group under the ATP-III guidelines. In contrast, the number of adults 40 to 59 years of age eligible for primary prevention therapy is similar between the two guidelines, which suggests that age has a greater impact than other risk factors in the new risk assessment models to such an extent that older men can be encouraged to start statin therapy based on age alone.

RISK ASSESSMENT EQUATIONS

The National Cholesterol Education Program's updated clinical guidelines on the Detection, Evaluation, and Treatment of High Blood Cholesterol in Adults (ATP-III) were published in 2001 and are now widely used by physicians to assess, manage, and follow up patients.[7] These guidelines place strong emphasis on the primary prevention of CVD in adults with multiple risk factors. A calculator to assess the 10-year risk for MI and coronary death (hard CHD) was developed by using data from the Framingham Heart Study. Risk status is determined by a 2-step procedure wherein presence/absence or level of risk factors are first counted giving a total point score from which a 10-year risk assessment is performed with a Framingham scoring sheet. Framingham scoring divides persons with multiple risk factors into those with 10-year risk for CHD of greater than 20%, 10% to 20%, and less than 10%. Intensity of treatment and goals of therapy are then decided based on the category into which that individual is placed (**Table 3**).

An update to the ATP-III guidelines[8] was published in July 2004 based on 5 statin trials: the Heart Protection Study (HPS), the Prospective Study of Pravastatin in the

Table 3
National Cholesterol Education Program Adult Treatment Panel III LDL-C goals for different risk categories

Risk Category	LDL Goal (mg/dL)	LDL Level at Which to Initiate Therapeutic Life Style Changes (mg/dL)	LDL Level at Which to Consider Drug Therapy (mg/dL)
0–1 risk factor	<160	≥160	≥190 (160–189: LDL-lowering drug optional)
2+ risk factors (10-y risk ≤20%)	<130	≥130	10-y risk 10%–20%: 130 10-y risk <10%: 160
CHD or CHD risk equivalents (10-y risk >20%)	<100	≥100	≥130 (100–129: drug optional)

Data from Expert Panel on Detection, Evaluation, and Treatment of High Blood Cholesterol in Adults. Executive summary of the third report of the National Cholesterol Education Program (NCEP) Expert Panel on Detection, Evaluation, and Treatment of High Blood Cholesterol in Adults (Adult Treatment Panel III). JAMA 2001;285(19):2486–97.

Elderly at Risk (PROSPER) study, Antihypertensive and Lipid-lowering Treatment to Prevent Heart Attack Trial Lipid-lowering Trial (ALLHAT-LLT), Anglo-Scandinavian Cardiac Outcomes Trial Lipid-lowering Arm (ASCOT-LLA), and the Pravastatin or Atorvastatin Evaluation and Infection Therapy (PROVE-IT) trial. The recommendation was made to lower LDL-C levels in very-high-risk patients to less than 70 mg/dL. These recommendations did not change the previous ATP-III calculation of risk (**Table 4**).

In 2008, D'Agostino and colleagues[9] proposed an expanded Framingham global CVD score as a more recent sex-specific multivariable calculator for use in the primary care setting for predicting the risk of developing a cardiac event. These more inclusive cardiac events were defined by adding angina, fatal and nonfatal stroke, TIA, claudication, and congestive heart failure to MI and CHD death, which were used in the 2001 and 2004 ATP-III calculators. The investigators evaluated 8491 Framingham study participants (mean age, 49 years; 4522 women) who attended a routine examination between 30 and 74 years of age and were free of CVD. The general CVD algorithm showed good discrimination (C-statistic, 0.763 [men] and 0.793 [women]) and calibration (χ^2, 13.48 in men and 7.79 for the women).

Several statistical criteria were used to assess performance of different risk equations in the new guidelines. A model is well calibrated if it correctly predicts the proportion of patients with given characteristics who develop disease. The modified Hosmer-Lemeshow χ^2 statistic was used for determining calibration. This statistic measures how well predicted and observed disease counts agree. A χ^2 value of greater than 20 or a P value of less than .05 indicates poor calibration, although these quantities depend on the sample size. A model has good discriminatory accuracy if the distribution of predicted risks is much higher in cases than in noncases. A popular measure of discriminatory accuracy is the C index: the probability that a randomly selected case will have a higher predicted risk than a randomly selected noncase. The ideal risk model would have a C index of 1.0; all cases would have predicted risks above a specific cut point value, and all noncases below it. This ideal rarely occurs. A C index between 0.70 and 0.80 is considered moderate to good and 0.80 or greater is considered excellent. The net reclassification index (NRI) measures the ability of a risk factor added to a previous predictive equation to accurately reclassify a person with an event into the stratified group of persons with events, and to accurately reclassify a person without an event into the stratified group of

Table 4
Adult Treatment Panel III and Adult Treatment Panel update guidelines for cholesterol goals

Risk Category	LDL Goal (mg/dL)	Initiate TLC (mg/dL)	Consider Drug Therapy (mg/dL)
Very high risk	<70 (optional)	≥70	≥70
High risk: 10-y risk >20%	<100	≥100	≥100
Moderately high risk: ≥2 risk factors 10-y risk 10%–20%	<130 <100 (optional)	≥130 ≥100 (optional)	≥130
Moderate risk: ≥2 risk factors 10-y risk <10%	<130	≥130	≥160
Low risk: 0–1 risk factor	<160	≥160	≥190

Data from Grundy SM, Cleeman JI, Bairey Merz CN, et al. Implications of recent clinical trials for the National Cholesterol Education Program Adult Treatment Panel III guidelines. J Am Coll Cardiol 2004;44(3):720–32. Available at: http://eresources.library.mssm.edu:2213/10.1016/j.jacc.2004.07.001.

persons without an event minus those who have been accurately classified and now are inaccurately classified.

The new 2013 ACC/AHA Guidelines for the Assessment of Cardiovascular Risk provide race-specific and sex-specific pooled cohort equations to:

1. Predict the 10-year risk for development of ASCVD in non-Hispanic white and African American men and women, 40 to 79 years of age, who are not receiving statin therapy, and who have untreated LDL-C levels of greater than or equal to 70 mg/dL to less than 190 mg/dL; and
2. Assess 30-year or lifetime ASCVD risk in adults 20 to 59 years of age without ASCVD and who are not at high short-term risk

In July 2012, the American Stroke Association[10] called for the inclusion of atherosclerotic stroke along with MI and sudden cardiac death as a high-risk condition and as a cardiovascular event outcome in risk prediction algorithms for vascular disease in order to better identify patients who may benefit from preventive measures. Thus, in contrast with the 2008 Framingham model described earlier, the newly developed risk prediction algorithms expanded the scope of prevention from a more general CVD to hard ASCVD events, including the risk of nonfatal MI, CHD death, and nonfatal and fatal stroke. Revascularization events in the 2008 global CVD score that tend to be influenced by provider preference and those with poor reliability, such as angina and congestive heart failure, were left out of the outcomes.

The new guidelines recommend initiation of statin therapy for primary prevention in patients with predicted 10-year risks of greater than or equal to 7.5%, and consideration of statin therapy in patients with 10-year risks of between 5% and 7.5%. In patients with diabetes, the threshold of greater than or equal to 7.5% can be used to select between high-intensity and moderate-intensity statin regimens.

The new equations apply to non-Hispanic African and non-Hispanic white Americans to predict the 10-year risk of developing a first hard ASCVD event. Because these equations do not include Hispanic white, Asian, and Indian Americans, the Guidelines recommend using the equations for the non-Hispanic white population, with a caution that there might be an overestimation of risk in the Hispanic white population and an underestimation of risk in American Indians.

DEVELOPING THE NEW AMERICAN COLLEGE OF CARDIOLOGY/AMERICAN HEART ASSOCIATION POOLED COHORT 10-YEAR RISK EQUATION

The ACC/AHA Work Group decided to develop new equations for 10-year risk assessment rather than use preexisting algorithms.[11] The decision to do so was based on concerns that the existing risk equations (1) were not able to be generalized to nonwhite community-based cohorts, (2) had narrow end points of hard CHD not accounting for stroke and other atherosclerotic events, (3) did not include diabetes mellitus in the multivariable risk equations, and (4) did not consider novel risk factors beyond the traditional risk factors. Pooled data from 5 community-based, National Heart, Lung and Blood Institute–funded, epidemiologic cohorts of African American and non-Hispanic white men and women with greater than 12 years of follow-up were used to develop the new sex-specific and race-specific equations. These cohorts included the Atherosclerosis Risk in Communities (ARIC) study, the Cardiovascular Health Study (CHS), and the Coronary Artery Risk Development in Young Adults (CARDIA) study, in addition to the original Framingham Heart Study and its Offspring Cohorts Study (**Table 5**).

Table 5
Cohorts used to develop the new sex-specific and race-specific equations

Study	Race	Gender	Total (n)	Age (y)	Location	Total Cholesterol mM/L	Total Cholesterol mg/dL	HDL-C mM/L	HDL-C mg/dL	UnRx SBP (mm Hg)	Rx SBP (mm Hg)	Current Smoker (%)	Diabetes (%)	10-y ASCVD Rate (%)
Framingham, Framingham Offspring[46,47]	White	Female	3470	40–74	Framingham, MA	5.79	224	1.50	58	127	148	33	5	3.8
	White	Male	2995			5.61	217	1.16	45	130	146	34	8	9.5
ARIC[14]	White	Female	5508	44–65	Forsyth County, NC; Jackson, MS;	5.64	218	1.50	58	114	129	25	6	3.6
	White	Male	4692			5.43	210	1.11	43	118	129	25	8	9.0
	African American	Female	2137	44–66	Minneapolis, MN; Washington County, MD	5.59	216	1.50	58	124	133	24	17	7.2
	African American	Male	1364			5.46	211	1.32	51	128	134	37	15	11.1
CARDIA[13]	White	Female	131	40–42	Birmingham, AL; Chicago, IL;	4.68	181	1.40	54	105	108	18	2	0.0
	White	Male	103			4.80	186	1.11	43	113	114	23	3	1.0
	African American	Female	110	40–45	Minneapolis, MN; Oakland, CA	4.68	181	1.37	53	111	130	27	6	0.9
	African American	Male	64			4.84	187	1.22	47	117	128	38	3	4.7
CHS[12]	White	Female	2131	65–79	Forsyth County, NC; Sacramento County, CA;	5.77	223	1.55	60	130	141	13	10	18.0
	White	Male	1308			5.17	200	1.24	48	132	142	11	15	28.5
	African American	Female	394	65–79	Washington County, MD; Pittsburgh, PA	5.56	215	1.58	61	137	146	14	22	23.0
	African American	Male	219			5.17	200	1.34	52	134	144	24	26	24.9
Total			24,626											
	White	Female	11,240											
	White	Male	9098											
	African American	Female	2641											
	American	Male	1647											

Abbreviations: Rx SBP, treated systolic blood pressure; UnRx SBP, untreated systolic blood pressure.
Data from Refs.[12,14,15,46,47]

The CHS[12] was designed to identify risk factors for CHD and stroke in older adults greater than or equal to 65 years of age. In addition to measuring the usual risk factors, particular interest was taken in the measurement of subclinical atherosclerotic disease, which has increased prevalence in the elderly. The CARDIA study[13] was initiated to investigate cardiovascular risk factors in young adults 18 to 30 years of age. The ARIC study[14] was conducted to study the cause of atherosclerosis; its clinical sequelae; and variation in risk factors based on race, sex, place, and time in adults 45 to 64 years of age with a median follow-up of 10 years.

A total of 11,240 white women, 9098 white men, 2641 African American women, and 1647 African American men between the ages of 40 and 79 years and without a history of MI (recognized or unrecognized), stroke, congestive heart failure, percutaneous coronary intervention, coronary bypass surgery, or atrial fibrillation were included.

ASCVD risk estimates included the covariates of age, treated or untreated systolic blood pressure (SBP), total cholesterol, high-density lipoprotein cholesterol (HDL-C), current smoking, and diabetes. Additional risk factors like diastolic BP, family history of ASCVD, moderate or severe chronic kidney disease, and body mass index (BMI) were not included because none of them improved discrimination for 10-year risk prediction when added to the models. Other risk factors like hs-CRP, apolipoprotein B, microalbuminuria, cardiorespiratory fitness, CAC, carotid intimal-medial thickness (CIMT), and ABI were also not included for lack of data because these risk factors and measures of ASCVD were not included in the examined cycles of the studies.

Using the new pooled 10-year risk equations on the 5 populations from which they were derived, internal validation results yielded C-statistics of 0.805 for white women, 0.746 for white men, 0.818 for African American women, and 0.713 for African American men. As seen from the C-statistics, these equations have a good to excellent ability to discriminate in the derivation cohort those who will experience a hard ASCVD event from those who will not.

External validation was performed in 3 populations: the Multi-Ethnic Study of Atherosclerosis (MESA) with a 6-year follow-up; Reasons for Geographic and Racial Differences in Stroke (REGARDS) with a 4-year follow-up; and in the most contemporary data available from ARIC, Framingham original, and Framingham Offspring with a 10-year follow-up. C-statistics ranged from 0.56 (African American men in the REGARDS cohort) to 0.77 (African American women in the MESA cohort). In the 12 cohorts studied (African American and white men and women in the 3 study populations), C-statistics were greater than 0.7 in 6 of 12 cohorts, more than 0.65 in 4 of 12 cohorts, and less than 0.6 in 2 of 12 cohorts. The pooled cohort equations tend to overestimate risk; less so in the lower risk, more so in the higher risk categories (see Table 7 of the Full Work Group Report supplement,[15] http://jaccjacc.cardiosource.com/acc_documents/2013_FPR_S5_Risk_Assessment.pdf)

ASSESSING THE NEW AMERICAN COLLEGE OF CARDIOLOGY/AMERICAN HEART ASSOCIATION POOLED COHORT 10-YEAR RISK EQUATION

Since the release of the new calculator, clinicians have questioned the accuracy of its clinical predictions. Part of the controversy relates to uncertainty in the number of new people who would require statin therapy under these new guidelines. Risk estimators must predict event risk, which closely matches observed risk in populations other than those used for calculating the equations.

Using 3 large-scale primary prevention cohorts (the Women's Health Study, the Physicians' Health Study, and the Women's Health Initiative Observational Study),

Ridker and Cook[16] observed overestimation of risk by 75% to 150% at all levels of 4 gender-specific and race-specific 10-year risk categories.

The investigators of the 2013 ACC/AHA Risk Assessment Guideline, Lloyd-Jones and colleagues defended their position to lower the treatment threshold to 7.5%, which would still provide a buffer with the treatment threshold of 5% shown in trials to provide clinical benefit. Their risk equations overestimate risk mainly in high-risk individuals for whom treatment decision may already have been made rather than low-risk individuals who do not need a statin. The investigators also point out that the 3 primary prevention cohorts used by Ridker and colleagues for their analysis comprised low-risk white populations with remarkably low event rates and hence are not representative of the US population.

REGARDS investigators Muntner and colleagues[17,18] suggest that it is premature to conclude that the new risk equations overestimate risk for the following reasons:

1. The contemporary nature of the MESA and REGARDS cohorts reflects improvements in overall health and lifestyle patterns in the United States over the past 25 years since observations in the original derivation cohort started.
2. In the most recent comparative cohorts, study participants may have been prescribed statins after enrollment based on their baseline test results, leading to altered long-term outcomes.
3. There has been an increased use of revascularization procedures, which can reduce the incidence of hard ASCVD events. Maximum overestimation of risk was therefore observed in the high-risk group.
4. Studies used to develop the risk equations included active surveillance(determining outcomes using periodic telephone calls, searching ASCVD diagnostic codes in the local hospital or regional death records, and documenting out-of-hospital ASCVD events by contact with family or physician) in addition to self-reporting of cardiovascular events. The lack of surveillance components in the contemporary validation studies could lead to under-reporting and be a reason for the overestimation of ASCVD incidence.

In a more recent publication, these same investigators[18] reevaluated the calibration and discrimination of the pooled cohort risk equations in the REGARDS cohort and in participants who could be considered for statin therapy (45–79 years of age, without clinical ASCVD or diabetes, with LDL-C levels between 70 and 189 mg/dL and not taking statins). The equations overestimate risk in the entire REGARDS study population but overestimation of risk was smaller in the subpopulation that would be considered for statin therapy. Further analysis was performed in subjects greater than or equal to 65 years of age who had Medicare claims data available (a form of active surveillance for ASCVD events). In this group the risk equations underestimated ASCVD events (**Table 6**).

RATIONALE FOR CONSTRUCTING MODELS TO ASSESS THE LONG-TERM/LIFETIME RISK FOR A FIRST HARD ATHEROSCLEROTIC CARDIOVASCULAR DISEASE EVENT

The short-term risk equations do not predict the lifetime risk of hard ASCVD events that develop as a result of increasing number or severity of risk factors. The increasing life expectancy of the population would translate into a higher incidence of ASCVD in an older population. Predicting an individual's lifetime risk of developing hard ASCVD events may hence serve in helping individuals decide whether to significantly change lifestyle or to start statins.

Studies of lifetime risk so far have been based on a variety of risk factor stratification strategies defined by categorical definition of risk factors: risk factor absence or

Table 6
Validation of the 10-year risk prediction equations in the REGARDS data

10-y ASCVD Risk (%)	Observed 5-y Incidence Rate/1000 Patient Years	Predicted 5-y Incidence Rate/1000 Patient Years	Calibration Hosmer-Lemeshow χ^2 >20 Poor	Discrimination C-Statistic Moderate–Good (0.70–0.79)
Overall Population (N = 18,498)				
5 to <7.5	4.2	4.8	84.2	0.71
7.5 to <10	5.0	6.8		
≥10	12.6	17.8		
Subgroup for Statin Consideration: No ASCVD, No Diabetes and LDL-C Level 70–189 mg/dL (N = 10,997)				
5 to <7.5	4.8	4.8	19.9	0.72
7.5 to <10	6.1	6.9		
≥10	12	15.1		
Medicare Linked Data (N = 6121)				
<7.5	5.3	4.1	11.4	0.65
7.5 to <10	7.7	6.5		
≥10	18.2	19.3		
Medicare Subgroup for Statin Consideration: No ASCVD, No Diabetes and LDL-C Level 70–189 mg/dL (N = 3333)				
<7.5	5.3	4	5.4	0.71
7.5 to <10	7.9	6.4		
≥10	17.4	16.4		

Data from Muntner P, Colantonio LD, Cushman M, et al. Validation of the atherosclerotic cardiovascular disease pooled cohort risk equations. JAMA 2014;311(14):1406–15. http://dx.doi.org/10.1001/jama.2014.2630.

presence (smoking, diabetes) and 3 to 4 risk factor levels of SBP (including or not including diastolic blood pressure [DBP]) and total cholesterol, HDL-C, and treatment or not of hypertension (treatment means higher lifetime risk, presumably because blood pressure has been higher for longer and thus on-treatment status adds risk to that reported by measured blood pressure level alone). Ten studies were identified with a follow-up of more than 15 years that provided long-term outcomes data in individuals at low or intermediate short-term risk. These studies have shown that young individuals, who have low 10-year predicted risk for CHD despite having a significant risk factor burden, are at a very high risk for developing CHD over their remaining lifespans.[19,20]

The long-term risk assessment for ASCVD is recommended for adults aged 20 to 39 years with LDL-C less than 190 mg/dL and adults 40 to 59 years of age who are free from ASCVD and at low 10-year risk less than 7.5%, not at 10-year risk greater than or equal to 7.5%. The investigators of the new guidelines noted that the Framingham 10-year risk score could not be used to predict lifetime risk because extrapolation from 10-year risk scores underestimate the observed lifetime risk. The lifetime risk score that was developed was able to stratify CHD lifetime risk fairly well in women of all ages but not as well in young men. For example, a 40-year-old woman in the lowest, middle, and highest tertiles of predicted 10-year CHD risk, the remaining lifetime risks for CHD to age 84 years were 12.2%, 25.4%, and 33.2%, respectively. In contrast, the lifetime risks for a 40-year-old man were 38.4%, 41.7%, and 50.7%, respectively.[21]

Pencina and colleagues[22] compared the 10-year and lifetime risks for ASCVD events, and prospectively followed 4506 participants of the Framingham Offspring cohort aged 20 to 59 years and free of CVD at baseline for the development of hard CVD events (coronary death, MI, and fatal and nonfatal stroke). Participants were followed for a maximum of 35 years. The investigators compared the results of 30-year risk estimates obtained by diverse methods: (1) tripling a 10-year risk estimate without accounting for the competing risks (naive approach); (2) estimating 3 event probabilities for each person with the 10-year risk calculators using the baseline age, age plus 10 years, and age plus 20 years, while maintaining the same baseline risk factor levels in all 3 models (combined approach), and calculating the 30-year risk as 1 minus the product of these three 10-year probabilities; (3) a 30-year risk estimate not accounting for competing risks (unadjusted approach); and (4) a 30-year risk estimate accounting for competing risks (adjusted approach). Long-term or lifetime risk estimation models adjusting for competing causes of mortality were shown to be more valid than extrapolation of results from 10-year risk equations.

For the lifetime risk equations in the new guidelines, Lloyd-Jones and colleagues[15] followed 3564 men and 4362 women enrolled in the Framingham Heart and Offspring Study who were free of CVD (MI, coronary insufficiency, angina, stroke, claudication) at 50 years of age. Lifetime risks were estimated to 95 years of age with non-CVD death as a competing event. Compared with participants with greater than or equal to 2 major risk factors, those with optimal levels had substantially lower lifetime risks (5.2% vs 68.9% in men, 8.2% vs 50.2% in women). For a comparative view of the stratified risk factors used in developing the lifetime risk equations and how increasing level of risk factors affects lifetime risk see **Table 7**. Individuals age ≥ 50 years who have a lifetime ASCVD risk double the 10 year coronary-equivalent risk of ≥ 20% would have a high lifetime risk ≥ 40% which is present in 60% of Framingham participants that age. **Table 7** may be helpful in physician/patient understanding of the importance and significance of lifetime risk for middle-aged patients. For other ages, lifetime risk for those in the lowest risk category is given, allowing a discussion

Table 7
Short-term and lifetime ASCVD risk in Framingham subjects aged ≥ 50 years

Risk Category	Subjects (%)	10-y ASCVD Risk (%)	Lifetime ASCVD Risk (M + F) (%)	Lifetime ASCVD Risk: M (%)	Lifetime ASCVD Risk: F (%)
≥2 Major risk factors: TC ≥240 mg/dL, SBP ≥160 mm Hg, DBP ≥100 mm Hg, DM, current smoking	20	10–25	>50	68.9	50.2
1 Major risk factor	40	10	39–50	50.4	38.8
≥1 Increased risk factors: TC 200–239 mg/dL, SBP 140–159 mm Hg, DBP 90–99 mm Hg, no DM, no smoking	23	5	39–46	45.5	39.1
≥1 Nonoptimal risk factors: TC 180–199 mg/dL, SBP 120–139 mm Hg, DBP 80–89 mm Hg, no DM, no smoking	12	<5	27–36	36.4	26.9
Optimal risk factors: TC <180 mg/dL, SBP <120 mm Hg, DBP <80 mm Hg, no DM, no smoking	4	<5	<10	5.2	8.2

Abbreviation: TC, total cholesterol.
Data from Lloyd-Jones DM, Leip EP, Larson MG, et al. Prediction of lifetime risk for cardiovascular disease by risk factor burden at 50 years of age. Circulation 2006;113(6):791–8. http://dx.doi.org/10.1161/CIRCULATIONAHA.105.548206.

with the patient of what lifestyle they may want to change or whether they want to take statins to lower increased lifetime risk.

Because the data for the current lifetime risk estimates are from the Framingham Heart and Offspring Study participants, risks calculated are derived from a non-Hispanic white population. Newer lifetime risk calculators will be forthcoming as reviewed in a meta-analysis of lifetime risks of hard ASCVD events from approximately 250,000 participants (including African Americans) from 18 long-term cohort studies published in 2012.[23]

The investigators of the new guidelines found that lifetime risk equations predicted CHD death with good discrimination (0.76–0.81 women and 0.71–0.75 in men). Pencina and colleagues[22] previously showed that lifetime risk equations have an improved validity when ASCVD risk factors are updated every 4 to 6 years and this is what the new guidelines suggest in terms of periodic reassessment of risk.

The 10-year and lifetime risk calculators can be downloaded at http://my.ame ricanheart.org/cvriskcalculator and http://www.cardiosource.org/en/Science-And-Quality/Practice-Guidelines-and-Quality-Standards/2013-Prevention-Guideline-Tools. aspx (**Fig. 1**).

Also, examples of 10-year and lifetime risk in a 55-year-old white man and woman with total cholesterol of 213 mg/dL, HDL-C 50 mg/dL, untreated SBP of 120 mm Hg, no diabetes, and no smoking are shown in **Fig. 2**.

OTHER MEASUREMENTS

The Work Group tested additional new markers for inclusion in the risk model. These markers included several blood and urine biomarkers (hs-CRP, apolipoprotein B, creatinine [or estimated glomerular filtration rate], and microalbuminuria), several measures of subclinical CVD (CAC, CIMT, ABI), family history, and cardiorespiratory fitness. Thirteen meta-analysis and systematic reviews including studies with at least 10 years of follow-up were reviewed. None of these markers have been evaluated as a screening test in RCTs with clinical events as outcomes. It is the opinion of the Work

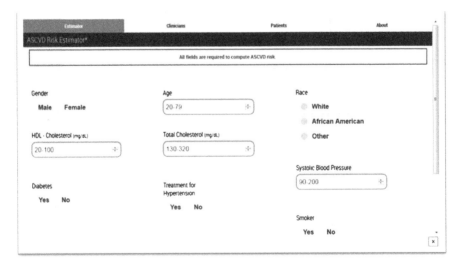

Fig. 1. Downloadable 2013 ASCVD risk calculator. (*From* American Heart Association. Available at: http://my.americanheart.org/professional/StatementsGuidelines/Prevention-Guidelines_UCM_457698_SubHomePage.jsp. Accessed August 13, 2014; with permission.)

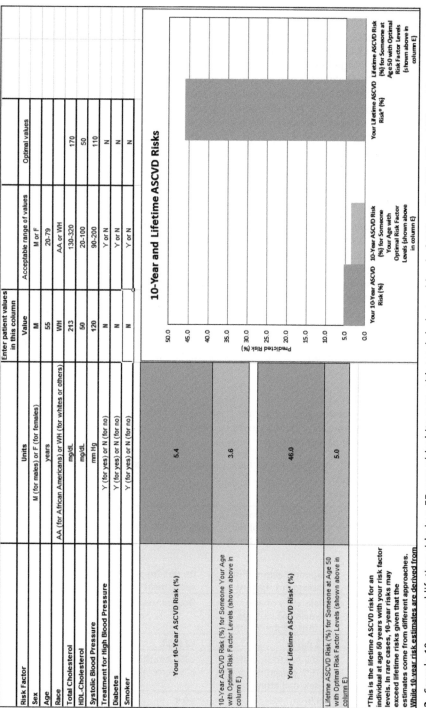

Risk Factor	Units	Enter patient values in this column		
		Value	Acceptable range of values	Optimal values
Sex	M (for males) or F (for females)	M	M or F	
Age	years	55	20–79	
Race	AA (for African Americans) or WH (for whites or others)	WH	AA or WH	
Total Cholesterol	mg/dL	213	130–320	170
HDL-Cholesterol	mg/dL	50	20–100	50
Systolic Blood Pressure	mm Hg	120	90–200	110
Treatment for High Blood Pressure	Y (for yes) or N (for no)	N	Y or N	N
Diabetes	Y (for yes) or N (for no)	N	Y or N	N
Smoker	Y (for yes) or N (for no)	N	Y or N	N

Your 10-Year ASCVD Risk (%)	5.4	
10-Year ASCVD Risk (%) for Someone Your Age with Optimal Risk Factor Levels (shown above in column E)	3.6	
Your Lifetime ASCVD Risk* (%)	46.0	
Lifetime ASCVD Risk (%) for Someone at Age 50 with Optimal Risk Factor Levels (shown above in column E)	5.0	

*This is the lifetime ASCVD risk for an individual at age 50 years with your risk factor levels. In rare cases, 10-year risks may exceed lifetime risks given that the estimates come from different approaches. While 10-year risk estimates are derived from

Fig. 2. Sample 10-year and lifetime risks in a 55-year-old white man with total cholesterol level of 213 mg/dL, HDL-C level 50 mg/dL, untreated SBP of 120 mm Hg, no diabetes, and not a smoker.

Group that assessments of family history of premature CVD and measurement of hs-CRP, CAC, and ABI show some promise for clinical utility among the novel risk markers, based on limited data (**Table 8**).

CAC reference values have been developed from the MESA study.[24] Participants were free of clinical CVD and treated diabetes at baseline. They were between 45 and 84 years of age, and identified themselves as white, African American, Hispanic, or Chinese. The calculator can be accessed at http://www.mesa-nhlbi.org/Calcium/input.aspx. The CAC score generated for an individual can be compared with others of the same age, gender, and race/ethnicity who do not have clinical CVD or treated diabetes. A systematic review by Peters and colleagues[25] reported NRI ranging from 14% to 25% for CAC as opposed to −1.4% to 12% for CIMT and 8% to 11% for carotid plaques. Uncertainty remains regarding assessing CAC because:

1. Most studies have assessed CHD outcomes and not hard ASCVD events
2. Widespread CAC screening would increase the risk of radiation exposure and the costs incurred

CAC has been proposed as a class IIb recommendation for individuals at moderate risk for whom a risk-based treatment decision is uncertain. Statin therapy can be initiated in the presence of a significant CAC (≥300 Agatston units or >75th percentile for age/gender group).

ABI can easily be assessed in routine practice and a value of less than 0.9 might support initiation of treatment. In a recently published meta-analysis of CIMT, Den Ruijter and colleagues[26] reported only a small net reclassification improvement of 0.8% (95% confidence interval [CI], 0.1%–1.6%) in 10-year risk prediction of first-time MI or stroke. Problems with CIMT measurement standardization led the Work Group to recommend against use of CIMT in routine medical practice.

STATIN SAFETY

The guidelines recommend moderate-dose statins rather than high-dose statins in individuals for whom high doses would be recommended because of the possibility of adverse effects of high dosage:

1. Individuals with multiple or serious comorbidities, including impaired renal or hepatic function

Table 8
Expert opinion thresholds for use of optional screening tests when risk-based decisions regarding initiation of pharmacologic therapy are uncertain following quantitative risk assessment

Measure	Support Revising Risk Assessment Upward	Do Not Support Revising Risk Assessment
Family history of premature CVD	Male <55 y of age Female <65 y of age (first-degree relative)	Occurrences at older ages only (if any)
hs-CRP	≥2 mg/L	<2 mg/L
CAC score	≥300 Agatston units or ≥75th percentile for age, sex, and ethnicity[a]	<300 Agatston units and <75 percentile for age, sex, and ethnicity[a]
ABI	<0.9	≥0.9

[a] For additional information, see http://www.mesa-nhlbi.org/CACReference.aspx.

2. Individuals with a history of previous statin intolerance or muscle disorders
3. Individuals with unexplained ALT increases greater than 3 times the upper limit of normal (ULN)
4. Individuals who use drugs that affect statin metabolism
5. Individuals who are more than 75 years of age

For those of Asian ancestry a lower dose statin at the start of statin therapy may be chosen.

For those with a hemorrhagic stroke, moderate-dose statins may be more appropriate, although on meta-analyses in the trials of more versus less statin there was no significant increase in hemorrhagic stroke (Relative risk [RR], 1.21; 95% CI, 0.85–1.17; P = .3). In the same meta-analysis in trials of statin versus placebo, there was no significant increase in hemorrhagic stroke (RR, 1.15; 95% CI, 0.93–1.41; P = .2) and ischemic stroke incidence was decreased by 20% (RR, 0.80; 95% CI, 0.74–0.87; P = .0001).[27]

A baseline ALT level was measured in the RCTs with statins and is recommended by the guidelines. Patients with increased ALT levels (usually >1.5–2 times the ULN) were excluded from statin trials and manufacturers state that unexplained ALT greater than 3 times the ULN is a contraindication to statin therapy. In RCTs increases in transaminase levels occur at equal rates in subjects on statins and subjects on placebo. No cases of hepatic failure were reported. Thus no follow-up ALT level is necessary unless a person develops symptoms of liver disease, which the guidelines list as fatigue, weakness, loss of appetite, abdominal pain, or significant yellowing of sclera, skin, or urine.

For patients who are concerned about statins as a cause of cancer, the meta-analysis of 170,000 persons in statin randomized trials showed that statins did not increase the incidence of total cancer (RR, 1.00; 95% CI, 0.96–1.04; P = .9), site-specific cancer, or the risk of cancer death.[27]

Statins can produce adverse muscle symptoms in 1% to 5% of subjects in controlled clinical trials and at higher frequencies in observational cohorts such as the one done in France of 8000 outpatients taking high-dose statin, in which muscular symptoms were reported in 10.5% of patients with a median time of onset of 1 month after statin initiation.[28] The management of these patients includes stopping the problematic statin and then rechallenging with a second statin. The Cleveland Clinic showed that 72.5% of intolerant patients were ultimately able to tolerate some regimen of long-term statin therapy.[29] They also used intermittent statin dosing rather than daily dosing in many patients and, although it did not produce as much LDL-C lowering, it nevertheless was better than no statin therapy. Other LDL-C–lowering drugs may be added, such as ezetimibe[30] and bile acid binders, to lower the LDL-C level further but there are no combination studies showing efficacy in reducing ASCVD events. Rhabdomyolysis occurs rarely (<0.06% over a mean treatment period of 4.8 to 5.1 years). A rate of creatine kinase increase greater than 3 times ULN occurs infrequently and at a similar rate in those treated with intensive-dose or moderate-dose statin therapy (0.02% for moderate-dose statin to 0.1% for higher dose statin) over a 1-year to 5-year treatment period.

The guidelines recommend a baseline history of muscle symptoms and, for patients with a family or personal history of muscle symptoms, a baseline CPK is recommended before starting statins. Follow-up CPK levels are not recommended unless a person develops significant muscle symptoms on statins, including pain, tenderness, stiffness, cramping, weakness, or fatigue. Statins would then be stopped until symptoms are relieved. For severe muscle symptoms, testing of CPK, creatinine, and urinalysis for myoglobinuria may be appropriate. Guidelines suggest restarting a patient on the same statin at the same or lower dose for establishment of causality. If symptoms reappear, another statin or use of intermittent day dosing of another statin might be tried. If there is no resolution of muscle symptoms after 2 months in patients stopping statins, a search for another cause should be instituted.

Many persons refuse statins because of a small risk of a diabetes diagnosis with statins compared with placebo. The following provides risk estimates that may be given to patients concerned about this unexplained small increased risk. A recent meta-analysis of 13 trials of statin therapy (including Justification for the Use of Statins in Prevention: An Intervention Trial Evaluating Rosuvastatin [JUPITER]) comparing statin versus placebo or usual care in 91,140 participants without diabetes reported an excess of 174 cases with new-onset diabetes (2226 vs 2052; Hazard Ratio, 1.09; 95% CI, 1.02–1.17).[31] There was no significant heterogeneity among statins, and the numbers needed to treat over 4 years to produce 1 new case of diabetes was 255, or 1 new case per 1000 treated per year compared with placebo. In the 150,000 women in the Women's Health Initiative, mean age 63 years and BMI of 28 kg/m^2, the cumulative incidence of diabetes over 9 years in the 7% of women on statins at years 1 and 3 versus those not on statins was 9.1% versus 6.0%, or an increased risk of diabetes of 3 per 100 over 9 years or 1 per 300 per year.[32] Highest dose statin therapy (atorvastatin 80 or simvastatin 80) versus lower dose statin therapy in 5 trials over 4 years involving 32,752 participants resulted in new-onset diabetes in 8.8% on statins versus 8.0% on moderate-dose statin therapy, or 1 extra case of new diabetes per 500 per year on the highest dose versus lower dose statin therapy. Meanwhile 3.2 CVD events were prevented per year.[33] In the JUPITER trial using Crestor 20 versus placebo for primary prevention in men more than 50 and women more than 60 years of age with LDL-C less than 130 mg/dL, and hs-CRP greater than or equal to 2, subjects without any risk factors for diabetes had no new-onset diabetes on Crestor versus placebo. In those on Crestor with 1 or more risk factors included in the metabolic syndrome, there was an absolute increase of 1 per 100 cases of diabetes but an absolute decrease of 2 per 100 ischemic CVD events.[34] For patients with diabetes, statins may increase hemoglobin A1c (HbA1c) from 0.1% to 0.3%,[35] although one meta-analysis showed no change in HbA1c in 26 statin trials ranging from 4 weeks to 4 years.[36]

The guidelines state and confirm that the potential for ASCVD risk reduction outweighs the risk of diabetes in all but those with the lowest ASCVD risk. Those who develop diabetes on a statin should be counseled on a healthy lifestyle, including achieving and maintaining a healthy body weight, participation in exercise, smoking cessation, and continuation of the statin to reduce the risk of an ASCVD event.

The panel did not find evidence that statins had an adverse effect on cognitive changes or risk of dementia. This finding has been confirmed in 2 recent meta-analyses.[37,38] The first cited a meta-analysis by Richardson and colleagues[38] who searched the US Food and Drug Administration database and found that the reported rates of cognitive-related adverse events were no higher for statins than for 2 drugs not know to cause cognitive impairment: losartan and clopidogrel (1.9 vs 1.6 and 1.9 per million written prescriptions). Thus the guidelines suggest that, for individuals presenting with a confusional state or memory impairment while on statin therapy, it may be reasonable to evaluate the patient for nonstatin causes, such as exposure to other drugs, as well as for systemic and neuropsychiatric causes in addition to the possibility of such an effect associated with statin drug therapy.

The National Lipid Association Task Force on Statin Safety Update 2014 has a supplement in the *Journal of Clinical Lipidology* that provides a more in-depth review of statin safety and management.[39]

SUMMARY

The 2013 ACC/AHA risk assessment and cholesterol treatment guidelines emphasize important core concepts and introduce new concepts for risk assessment. They differ substantially from the previous ATP-III guidelines, particularly with respect to primary prevention of CVD. The ATP-III guidelines place more emphasis on levels of LDL-C to select patients for statin therapy, whereas the new guidelines base the recommendation solely on the 10-year ASCVD predicted risk, as long as the LDL-C level is 70 to 189 mg/dL or higher. High-intensity statin treatment is recommended in all people with known ASCVD irrespective of their LDL-C levels and in those without such disease but at high LDL-C levels greater than or equal to 190 mg/dL or with diabetes with increased ASCVD risk. The guidelines have identified patient groups in which a more intensive treatment is superior to a moderate treatment, and focus on statins as the mainstay of therapy rather than clinically unproven lipid-lowering drug combinations. These steps are important to simplify and improve care for high-risk individuals. It is recommended that clinicians determine an individual's absolute 10-year risk score by standard clinical testing in order to engage in a meaningful clinician-patient discussion regarding the potential for ASCVD risk reduction, treatment adverse effects, drug-drug interactions, and patient preferences. The recommendation to treat individuals with 10-year risks of 7.5% or greater has been boosted by the newest validation study of REGARDS[18]; the validity of lifetime risk prediction algorithms remain controversial but may help in stimulating more serious conversations between doctors and patients at younger ages when 10-year risk is low. According to these new guidelines, more than 30 million people without existing CVD might be candidates for statin therapy. These large numbers should mobilize the medical community to identify potentially modifiable risk factors affected by lifestyle and institute behavioral changes before starting statins in order to further contain the epidemic of CVD. They are intended to guide decision making but not replace clinical judgment.

REFERENCES

1. Go AS, Mozaffarian D, Roger VL, et al. Executive summary: heart disease and stroke statistics–2014 update: a report from the American Heart Association. Circulation 2014;129(3):399–410. http://dx.doi.org/10.1161/01.cir.0000442015.53336.12.
2. Gregg EW, Li Y, Wang J, et al. Changes in diabetes-related complications in the united states, 1990-2010. N Engl J Med 2014;370(16):1514–23. http://dx.doi.org/10.1056/NEJMoa1310799.
3. Kaufman HW, Blatt AJ, Huang X, et al. Blood cholesterol trends 2001-2011 in the United States: analysis of 105 million patient records. PLoS One 2013;8(5):e63416. http://dx.doi.org/10.1371/journal.pone.0063416.
4. Stone NJ, Robinson JG, Lichtenstein AH, et al. 2013 ACC/AHA guideline on the treatment of blood cholesterol to reduce atherosclerotic cardiovascular risk in adults: a report of the American College of Cardiology/American Heart Association Task Force on Practice Guidelines. J Am Coll Cardiol 2014;63(25 Pt B):2889–934. http://dx.doi.org/10.1016/j.jacc.2013.11.002.
5. Stone NJ, Robinson JG, Lichtenstein AH, et al. Treatment of blood cholesterol to reduce atherosclerotic cardiovascular disease risk in adults: synopsis of the 2013 American College of Cardiology/American Heart Association cholesterol guideline. Ann Intern Med 2014;160(5):339–43. http://dx.doi.org/10.7326/M14-0126.

6. Pencina MJ, Navar-Boggan AM, D'Agostino RB, et al. Application of new cholesterol guidelines to a population-based sample. N Engl J Med 2014;370(15): 1422–31. http://dx.doi.org/10.1056/NEJMoa1315665.

7. Expert Panel on Detection, Evaluation, and Treatment of High Blood Cholesterol in Adults. Executive summary of the third report of the National Cholesterol Education Program (NCEP) Expert Panel on Detection, Evaluation, and Treatment of High Blood Cholesterol in Adults (Adult Treatment Panel III). JAMA 2001; 285(19):2486–97.

8. Grundy SM, Cleeman JI, Bairey Merz CN, et al. Implications of recent clinical trials for the national cholesterol education program adult treatment panel III guidelines. J Am Coll Cardiol 2004;44(3):720–32.http://eresources.library.mssm. edu:2213/10.1016/j.jacc.2004.07.001.

9. D'Agostino RB, Vasan RS, Pencina MJ, et al. General cardiovascular risk profile for use in primary care: the Framingham Heart Study. Circulation 2008;117(6): 743–53. http://dx.doi.org/10.1161/CIRCULATIONAHA.107.699579.

10. Lackland DT, Elkind MS, D'Agostino RS, et al. Inclusion of stroke in cardiovascular risk prediction instruments: a statement for healthcare professionals from the American Heart Association/American Stroke Association. Stroke 2012;43(7): 1998–2027. http://dx.doi.org/10.1161/STR.0b013e31825bcdac.

11. Goff DC Jr, Lloyd-Jones DM, Bennett G, et al. 2013 ACC/AHA guideline on the assessment of cardiovascular risk: a report of the American College of Cardiology/American Heart Association Task Force on Practice Guidelines. J Am Coll Cardiol 2014;63(25 Pt B):2935–59. http://dx.doi.org/10.1016/j.jacc.2013. 11.005.

12. Fried LP, Borhani NO, Enright P, et al. The cardiovascular health study: design and rationale. Ann Epidemiol 1991;1(3):263–76.

13. Friedman GD, Cutter GR, Donahue RP, et al. CARDIA: study design, recruitment, and some characteristics of the examined subjects. J Clin Epidemiol 1988; 41(11):1105–16. pii:0895-4356(88)90080-7.

14. Chambless LE, Folsom AR, Sharrett AR, et al. Coronary heart disease risk prediction in the Atherosclerosis Risk in Communities (ARIC) study. J Clin Epidemiol 2003; 56(9):880–90. pii:S0895435603000556.

15. Lloyd-Jones DM, Leip EP, Larson MG, et al. Prediction of lifetime risk for cardiovascular disease by risk factor burden at 50 years of age. Circulation 2006; 113(6):791–8. http://dx.doi.org/10.1161/CIRCULATIONAHA.105.548206.

16. Ridker PM, Cook NR. Statins: new American guidelines for prevention of cardiovascular disease. Lancet 2013;382(9907):1762–5. http://dx.doi.org/10.1016/ S0140-6736(13)62388-0.

17. Muntner P, Safford MM, Cushman M, et al. Comment on the reports of overestimation of ASCVD risk using the 2013 AHA/ACC risk equation. Circulation 2014;129(2):266–7. http://dx.doi.org/10.1161/CIRCULATIONAHA.113.007648.

18. Muntner P, Colantonio LD, Cushman M, et al. Validation of the atherosclerotic cardiovascular disease pooled cohort risk equations. JAMA 2014;311(14): 1406–15. http://dx.doi.org/10.1001/jama.2014.2630.

19. Lloyd-Jones DM, Wilson PW, Larson MG, et al. Lifetime risk of coronary heart disease by cholesterol levels at selected ages. Arch Intern Med 2003;163(16): 1966–72. http://dx.doi.org/10.1001/archinte.163.16.1966.

20. Marma AK, Berry JD, Ning H, et al. Distribution of 10-year and lifetime predicted risks for cardiovascular disease in US adults: findings from the National Health and Nutrition Examination Survey 2003 to 2006. Circ Cardiovasc Qual Outcomes 2010;3(1):8–14. http://dx.doi.org/10.1161/CIRCOUTCOMES.109.869727.

21. Lloyd-Jones DM, Wilson PW, Larson MG, et al. Framingham risk score and prediction of lifetime risk for coronary heart disease. Am J Cardiol 2004;94(1): 20–4. http://dx.doi.org/10.1016/j.amjcard.2004.03.023.

22. Pencina MJ, D'Agostino RB, Larson MG, et al. Predicting the 30-year risk of cardiovascular disease: the Framingham Heart Study. Circulation 2009;119(24): 3078–84. http://dx.doi.org/10.1161/CIRCULATIONAHA.108.816694.

23. Berry JD, Dyer A, Cai X, et al. Lifetime risks of cardiovascular disease. N Engl J Med 2012;366(4):321–9. http://dx.doi.org/10.1056/NEJMoa1012848.

24. McClelland RL, Chung H, Detrano R, et al. Distribution of coronary artery calcium by race, gender, and age: results from the Multi-ethnic Study of Atherosclerosis (MESA). Circulation 2006;113(1):30–7. pii:CIRCULATIONAHA.105.580696.

25. Peters SA, den Ruijter HM, Bots ML, et al. Improvements in risk stratification for the occurrence of cardiovascular disease by imaging subclinical atherosclerosis: a systematic review. Heart 2012;98(3):177–84. http://dx.doi.org/10.1136/heartjnl-2011-300747.

26. Den Ruijter HM, Peters SA, Anderson TJ, et al. Common carotid intima-media thickness measurements in cardiovascular risk prediction: a meta-analysis. JAMA 2012;308(8):796–803. http://dx.doi.org/10.1001/jama.2012.9630.

27. Cholesterol Treatment Trialists' (CTT) Collaboration, Baigent C, Blackwell L, Emberson J, et al. Efficacy and safety of more intensive lowering of LDL cholesterol: a meta-analysis of data from 170,000 participants in 26 randomised trials. Lancet 2010;376(9753):1670–81. http://dx.doi.org/10.1016/S0140-6736(10)61350-5.

28. Bruckert E, Hayem G, Dejager S, et al. Mild to moderate muscular symptoms with high-dosage statin therapy in hyperlipidemic patients–the PRIMO study. Cardiovasc Drugs Ther 2005;19(6):403–14. http://dx.doi.org/10.1007/s10557-005-5686-z.

29. Mampuya WM, Frid D, Rocco M, et al. Treatment strategies in patients with statin intolerance: the Cleveland Clinic experience. Am Heart J 2013;166(3):597–603. http://dx.doi.org/10.1016/j.ahj.2013.06.004.

30. Ballantyne CM, Houri J, Notarbartolo A, et al. Effect of ezetimibe coadministered with atorvastatin in 628 patients with primary hypercholesterolemia: a prospective, randomized, double-blind trial. Circulation 2003;107(19):2409–15. http://dx.doi.org/10.1161/01.CIR.0000068312.21969.C8.

31. Sattar N, Preiss D, Murray HM, et al. Statins and risk of incident diabetes: a collaborative meta-analysis of randomised statin trials. Lancet 2010;375(9716): 735–42. http://dx.doi.org/10.1016/S0140-6736(09)61965-6.

32. Culver AL, Ockene IS, Balasubramanian R, et al. Statin use and risk of diabetes mellitus in postmenopausal women in the Women's Health Initiative. Arch Intern Med 2012;172(2):144–52. http://dx.doi.org/10.1001/archinternmed.2011.625.

33. Preiss D, Seshasai SR, Welsh P, et al. Risk of incident diabetes with intensive-dose compared with moderate-dose statin therapy: a meta-analysis. JAMA 2011; 305(24):2556–64. http://dx.doi.org/10.1001/jama.2011.860.

34. Ridker PM, Pradhan A, MacFadyen JG, et al. Cardiovascular benefits and diabetes risks of statin therapy in primary prevention: an analysis from the JUPITER trial. Lancet 2012;380(9841):565–71. http://dx.doi.org/10.1016/S0140-6736(12)61190-8.

35. Maki KC, Ridker PM, Brown WV, et al. An assessment by the statin diabetes safety task force: 2014 update. J Clin Lipidol 2014;8(Suppl 3):S17–29. http://dx.doi.org/10.1016/j.jacl.2014.02.012.

36. Zhou Y, Yuan Y, Cai RR, et al. Statin therapy on glycaemic control in type 2 diabetes: a meta-analysis. Expert Opin Pharmacother 2013;14(12):1575–84. http://dx.doi.org/10.1517/14656566.2013.810210.

37. Swiger KJ, Manalac RJ, Blumenthal RS, et al. Statins and cognition: a systematic review and meta-analysis of short- and long-term cognitive effects. Mayo Clin Proc 2013;88(11):1213–21. http://dx.doi.org/10.1016/j.mayocp.2013.07.013.

38. Richardson K, Schoen M, French B, et al. Statins and cognitive function: a systematic review. Ann Intern Med 2013;159(10):688–97. http://dx.doi.org/10.7326/0003-4819-159-10-201311190-00007.

39. Jacobson TA. NLA task force on statin safety–2014 update. J Clin Lipidol 2014; 8(Suppl 3):S1–4. http://dx.doi.org/10.1016/j.jacl.2014.03.003.

40. Randomised trial of cholesterol lowering in 4444 patients with coronary heart disease: The Scandinavian Simvastatin Survival Study (4S). Lancet 1994;344(8934): 1383–9.

41. Heart Protection Study Collaborative Group. MRC/BHF heart protection study of cholesterol lowering with simvastatin in 20,536 high-risk individuals: a randomised placebo-controlled trial. Lancet 2002;360(9326):7–22. pii:S0140-6736(02) 09327-3.

42. LaRosa JC, Grundy SM, Waters DD, et al. Intensive lipid lowering with atorvastatin in patients with stable coronary disease. N Engl J Med 2005;352(14):1425–35. pii:NEJMoa050461.

43. Sever PS, Dahlof B, Poulter NR, et al. Prevention of coronary and stroke events with atorvastatin in hypertensive patients who have average or lower-than-average cholesterol concentrations, in the Anglo-Scandinavian Cardiac Outcomes Trial– Lipid Lowering Arm (ASCOT-LLA): a multicentre randomised controlled trial. Lancet 2003;361(9364):1149–58. pii:S0140-6736(03)12948-0.

44. Colhoun HM, Betteridge DJ, Durrington PN, et al. Primary prevention of cardiovascular disease with atorvastatin in type 2 diabetes in the Collaborative Atorvastatin Diabetes Study (CARDS): multicentre randomised placebo-controlled trial. Lancet 2004;364(9435):685–96. http://dx.doi.org/10.1016/S0140-6736(04) 16895-5.

45. Ridker PM, Danielson E, Fonseca FA, et al. Rosuvastatin to prevent vascular events in men and women with elevated C-reactive protein. N Engl J Med 2008;359(21):2195–207. http://dx.doi.org/10.1056/NEJMoa0807646.

46. Dawber TR, Kannel WB, Lyell LP. An approach to longitudinal studies in a community: the Framingham Study. Ann N Y Acad Sci 1963;107:539–56.

47. Kannel WB, Feinleib M, McNamara PM, et al. An investigation of coronary heart disease in families. The Framingham Offspring Study. Am J Epidemiol 1979; 110(3):281–90.

Coronary Artery Calcium Scanning

The Key to the Primary Prevention of Coronary Artery Disease

Harvey S. Hecht, MD, FACC, FSCCT

KEYWORDS

- Calcium scanning • Atherosclerosis • Coronary artery disease

KEY POINTS

- The potential impact of coronary artery calcium scanning (CAC) on primary prevention cannot be overestimated because it eliminates the guesswork implicit in extrapolating risk from guidelines derived from large population bases to individual patients and provides a snapshot of the cumulative effect of an individual's life on the coronary circulation.
- The role of risk factors is most important in identifying treatable therapeutic targets after risk has been established by a test that is 100% specific for atherosclerosis and far superior to any risk factor–based paradigm.
- The remaining barriers include physician education to overcome instinctive clinging to the old established paradigms, patient education to increase awareness of the widespread availability and low radiation of CAC, and more widespread insurance reimbursement.

INTRODUCTION

Despite the overwhelming peer reviewed data supporting the role of CAC in the primary prevention of coronary artery disease (CAD), its penetration into clinical practice has been inexplicably low. Screening for lung, breast, and colon cancer has been officially endorsed by the US Preventive Services Task Force, whereas CAD, which kills more than all cancers combined, is not likely to be approved for screening by CAC in the near future. Instead, reliance is placed on risk assessment by various risk factor–based paradigms, all of which have proved inferior to CAC. **Fig. 1** illustrates the essential flaw in risk factor–based evaluations. In more than half a million patients presenting with their first myocardial infarction, almost half had less than 2 risk factors and 80% had less than or equal to 2. Moreover, mortality was inversely related to the number of risk factors.[1]

Disclosure/Conflict of Interest Statement: Philips Medical Systems consultant.
Department of Cardiology, Mount Sinai Medical Center, Icahn School of Medicine at Mount Sinai, One Gustave L. Levy Place, Box 1030, New York, NY 10029-6574, USA
E-mail address: harvey.hecht@mountsinai.org

Endocrinol Metab Clin N Am 43 (2014) 893–911
http://dx.doi.org/10.1016/j.ecl.2014.08.007
0889-8529/14/$ – see front matter © 2014 Elsevier Inc. All rights reserved.

RF: hypertension, smoking, dyslipidemia, diabetes, and FH (<60)
542,008 patients with first MI

| | # RF | | | | | |
	0	1	2	3	4	5
N	14.4%	34.1%	31.6%	15.4%	4.1%	0.4%
Age	71.5	68.6	64.	61.7	58.8	56.7
Hosp Mortality	14.9%	10.9%	7.9%	5.3%	4.2%	3.6%

Mortality OR 1.54: inverse # RF

"The high prevalence of the same risk factors mong patients without CHD decreases the discriminatory power of these risk factors to accurately predict which patients will develop MI or even clinically significant atherosclerosis."

Fig. 1. The number of risk factors and mortality in patients with first MI. MI, myocardial infarction; OR, odds ratio; RF, risk factors. (*Reproduced with permission* of Wiley from Hecht HS, Narula J. Coronary artery calcium scanning in asymptomatic patients with diabetes mellitus: A paradigm shift. J Diab 2012;4:342–50.)

THE CORONARY ARTERY CALCIUM SCAN

CAC is a noncontrast, limited chest CT scan acquired with an approximate 3- to 5-second breath hold that automatically quantitates calcified coronary plaque, providing both an absolute Agatston unit (AU) score and a percentile normalized for age, gender, and ethnicity. Radiation exposure has progressively declined to approximately 1 mSv, comparable to mammography (0.8 mSv). Newer reconstruction algorithms decrease this dose to approximately 0.5 mSv. Examples of CAC scans displaying varying degrees of plaque are displayed in **Fig. 2.**

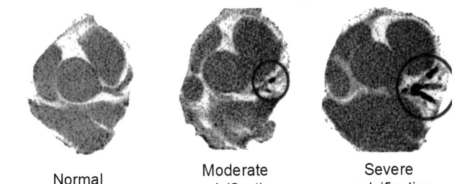

| Normal | Moderate calcification | Severe calcification |

Fig. 2. Examples of coronary artery scans.

THE PROGNOSTIC DATA

Every prognostic study, whether prospective or retrospective, population-based, or self-referred, has demonstrated the power of CAC, with relative risks (**Table 1**) far exceeding all risk factors, whether individually or collectively, in risk factor–based paradigms.[2–17]

Moreover, CAC has consistently added to the receiver operating characteristic (ROC) curve for risk factors and has always been superior to risk factors by themselves (**Fig. 3**).

Amalgamation of data from 5 large prospective randomized studies[9,11,14–16] yields 10-year event rates that can be translated into Framingham Risk Score (FRS) equivalents (**Table 2**).

Table 1
The prognostic power of coronary artery calcium in asymptomatic patients

	N	Mean Age (y)	Follow-up (y)	Calcium Score Cutoff	Comparator Group for RR Calculat	Relative Risk Ratio
Arad et al,[2] 2000	1173	53	3.6	CAC >160	CAC <160	20.2
Park et al,[3] 2002	967	67	6.4	CAC >142.1	CAC <3.7	4.9
Raggi et al,[4] 2000	632	52	2.7	Top quartile	Lowest quartile	13
Wong et al,[5] 2000	926	54	3.3	Top quartile (>270)	First quartile	8.8
Kondos et al,[6] 2003	5635	51	3.1	CAC	No CAC	10.5
Greenland et al,[7] 2004	1312	66	7.0	CAC >300	No CAC	3.9
Shaw et al,[8] 2003	10,377	53	5	CAC ≥400	CAC ≤10	8.4
Arad et al,[9] 2005	5585	59	4.3	CAC ≥100	CAC <100	10.7
Taylor et al,[10] 2005	2000	40–50	3.0	CAC >44	CAC = 0	11.8
Vliegenthart et al,[11] 2002	1795	71	3.3	CAC >1000 CAC 400–1000	CAC <100 CAC <100	8.3 4.6
Budoff et al,[12] 2007	25,503	56	6.8	CAC >400	CAC 0	9.2
Lagoski et al,[13] 2007	3601	45–84	3.75	CAC >0	CAC 0	6.5
Becker et al,[14] 2008	1726	57.7	3.4	CAC >400	CAC 0	6.8 Men 7.9 Women
Detrano et al,[15] 2008	6814	62.2	3.8	CAC >300	CAC 0	14.1
Erbel et al,[16] 2010	4487	45–75	5	>75th %	<25th %	11.1 Men 3.2 Women
Taylor et al,[17] 2010	1634	42	5.6	CAC >0	CAC 0	9.3

Reproduced with permission of Wiley from Hecht HS, Narula J. Coronary artery calcium scanning in asymptomatic patients with diabetes mellitus: A paradigm shift. J Diab 2012;4:342–50; and *Data from* Refs.[2,3,5–17]

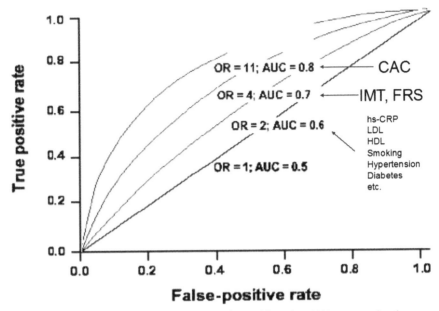

Fig. 3. The ROC curve, its AUC, and corresponding odds ratios. AUC, area under the curve; HDL, high-density lipoprotein; OR, odds ratio.

CAC greater than 400 is a CAD equivalent, with 10-year event rates exceeding 20% in asymptomatic patients. The absence of calcified plaque conveys an extraordinarily low 10-year risk (1.1%–1.7%), irrespective of the number of risk factors (**Fig. 4**).[18]

Of critical importance is the net reclassification index (NRI) conferred by CAC in the asymptomatic population by 3 major prospective population-based studies (**Table 3**).[11,15,16] The percentage of patients with FRS risk estimate correctly reclassified by CAC based on outcomes ranged from 52% to 65.6% in the intermediate-risk population, 34% to 35.8% in the high-risk group, and 11.6% to 15% in the low-risk cohort, with NRIs for the entire study population from 19% to 25%.

Comparison of CAC in the intermediate-risk population with risk markers other than those included in the FRS revealed its overwhelming superiority to ankle-brachial index, brachial flow–mediated dilation, carotid intima media thickness (IMT), family history (FH) of premature CAD, and high-sensitivity C-reactive protein (hs-CRP) (**Fig. 5**).[19]

In addition, multiple blood biomarkers, including hs-CRP, interleukin 8, myeloperoxidase, B-type natriuretic peptide; and plasminogen activator type 1, did not add to the

Table 2		
Event rates of CAC scores in asymptomatic patients and their FRS equivalents		
CAC	10-y Event Rate (%)	FRS Risk
0	1.1–1.7	Very low
1–100	2.3–5.9	Low
100–400	12.8–16.4	Intermediate
>400	22.5–28.6	High
>1000	37	Very high

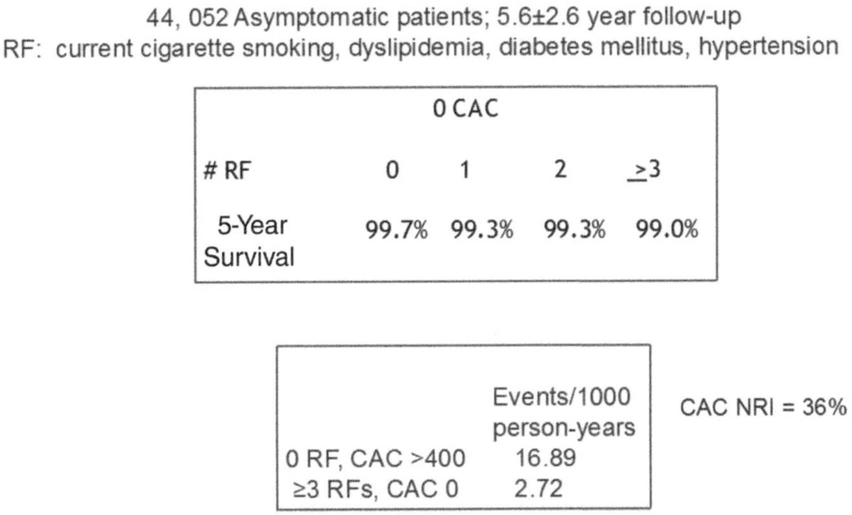

44, 052 Asymptomatic patients; 5.6±2.6 year follow-up
RF: current cigarette smoking, dyslipidemia, diabetes mellitus, hypertension

	0 CAC			
# RF	0	1	2	≥3
5-Year Survival	99.7%	99.3%	99.3%	99.0%

	Events/1000 person-years	
0 RF, CAC >400	16.89	CAC NRI = 36%
≥3 RFs, CAC 0	2.72	

Fig. 4. Interplay of CAC and traditional risk factors for prediction of all-cause mortality in asymptomatic patients. RF, risk factors. (*Data from* Nasir K, Rubin J, Blaha MJ, et al. Interplay of coronary artery calcification and traditional risk factors for the prediction of all-cause mortality in asymptomatic individuals. Circ Cardiovasc Imaging 2012;5:469.)

Table 3
Reclassification of FRS risk by CAC: primary prevention outcome studies

Study	Reclassified (%)	N	Age (y)	Follow-up (y)
MESA		5878	62.2	5.8
FRS 0%–6%	11.6			
FRS 6%–20%	54.4			
FRS >20%	35.8			
NRI	25			
Heinz Nixdorf		4487	45–75	5.0
FRS <10%	15.0			
FRS 10%–20%	65.6			
FRS >20%	34.2			
NRI	22.4			
Rotterdam		2028	69.6	9.2
FRS <10%	12			
FRS 10%–20%	52			
FRS >20%	34			
NRI	19			

Abbreviation: N, number of patients.
Reproduced with permission of Wiley from Hecht HS, Narula J. Coronary artery calcium scanning in asymptomatic patients with diabetes mellitus: A paradigm shift. J Diab 2012;4:342–50.

6814 MESA participants
1330 Intermediate FRS (5-20%) without DM
7.6-Year follow-up, 94 CHD, 123 CVD events

Risk Markers and CVD

Marker	Multivariate HR	P	NRI vs FRS
ABI	0.79	.01	.036
Brachial FMD	0.82	.52	.024
CAC	2.60	<.001	.659
Carotid IMT	1.33	.13	.102
Family history	2.18	.001	.160
hs-CRP	1.26	.05	.079

Fig. 5. Comparison of novel risk markers for improvement in cardiovascular risk assessment in intermediate-risk individuals. ABI, ankle-brachial index; CVD, cardiovascular disease; DM, diabetes mellitus; FMD, flow-mediated dilation; HR, hazard ratio. (*Data from* Okwuosa TM, Greenland P, Ning H, et al. Yield of screening for coronary artery calcium in early middle-age adults based on the 10-year Framingham risk score: The CARDIA Study. JACC Cardiovasc Imaging 2012;5(9):923–30.)

C statistic for CAD outcomes of CAC and the FRS, whereas CAC increased the FRS C statistic from 0.73 to 0.84 (**Fig. 6**).[20]

PATIENT SUBGROUPS
Inflammatory Diseases

Inflammation as the common pathway of atherosclerosis is one of the tenets of cardiovascular disease. Nonetheless, with the exception of diabetes mellitus, the focus of early identification of risk by CAC scanning has been on intermediate-risk patients irrespective of associated disease states. It is now clearly understood that cardiovascular risk is high and is often the leading cause of death in a broad spectrum of diseases with the common link of inflammation, which has been evaluated to varying degrees by CAC. There is sufficient evidence to warrant consideration of CAC scanning for patients with the inflammatory diseases shown in **Fig. 7** who may not otherwise be in the intermediate-risk category.

Diabetes

The 2010 American College of Cardiology Foundation (ACCF)/American Heart Association (AHA) Guideline for Assessment of Cardiovascular Risk in Asymptomatic Adults awarded a class IIa recommendation for all adults older than 40 with diabetes.[21] Although the initial reasoning was to identify the high-risk patients with CAC greater than 400 for further evaluation to rule out obstructive disease, CAC prognostic data have challenged the ingrained concept of diabetes mellitus as a CAD disease equivalent. Patients with diabetes and CAC have higher risks than those without diabetes and similar CAC, but the absence of CAC conveys a similar low risk in both groups (**Table 4**).[22–26] Therefore, the more appropriate rationale is for straightforward risk classification as with any other risk factor, allowing for the possibility of downgrading risk.

1,286 Asymptomatic patients (59 + 8 years)
Follow-up 4.1 y; 35 events

Biomarkers:
CRP
Interleukin 6
Myeloperoxidase
BNP
Plasminogen activator type 1

	c statistic	P
FRS	.73	
FRS + all bio	.75	.32
FRS + CAC	.84	.003
FRS + CAC + all bio	.84	NS

Fig. 6. Comparative value of CAC and multiple blood biomarkers for prognostication of cardiovascular events. BNP, beta natriuretic protein; CRP, C-reactive protein. (*Data from* Rana JS, Gransar H, Wong ND, et al. Comparative value of coronary artery calcium and multiple blood biomarkers for prognostication of cardiovascular events. Am J Cardiol 2012;109:1450.)

Family History of Premature Coronary Artery Disease

Many articles have documented the strong association between FH and both clinical and subclinical CAD.[27]

In the younger population (<45 for men and <55 for women), however, these patients are an overlooked higher-risk group who would not qualify for treatment based on the FRS or any other paradigm. In recognition of this problem, the 2009 CAC Appropriate Use Criteria[28,29] considered CAC "appropriate" for asymptomatic patients with an FH of premature CAD and a low global risk estimate. The best approach

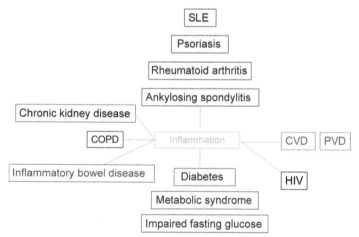

Fig. 7. Inflammatory diseases associated with a higher risk of CAD. COPD, chronic obstructive pulmonary disease; CVD, cardiovascular disease; PVD, peripheral vascular disease; SLE, systemic lupus erythematosis.

Table 4
Relationship between coronary artery calcium and events in asymptomatic diabetic patients

Study	N	Prevalence	Hazard Ratio	AUC	Event Rates/year
Wong et al,[22] 2003	1823	Any CAC No DM: 53% DM: 73.5%			0 CAC: 0.2% CAC >400: 5.6%
Becker et al,[23] 2008	716 DM	0 CAC: 15% CAC >400: 42%		CAC: 0.77 FRS: 0.68 UKPDS: 0.71 $P<.01$	
Elkeles et al,[24] 2008	589 DM		Compared with CAC 0–10 CAC >1000: 13.8 CAC 401–1000: 8.4 CAC 101–400: 7.1 CAC 11–100: 4.0	CAC: 0.73 UKPDS: 0.63 $P<.03$	CAC <10: 0%
Anand et al,[25] 2006	510 DM	CAC <10: 53.7%	Compared with CAC <100: CAC >1000: 58 CAC 401–1000: 41 CAC 101–400: 10	CAC: 0.92 UKPDS: 0.74 FRS: 0.60 $P<.001$	
Malik et al,[26] 2011	881 DM1 4036 No DM		Increasing CAC: 2.9–6.5 Increasing CAC: 2.6–9.5	CAC + RF: 0.78–0.80 RF: 0.72–0.73 $P<.001$	1.5% 0.5%

Abbreviations: AUC, area under curve; DM, diabetes mellitus.
Reproduced with permission of Wiley from Hecht HS, Narula J. Coronary artery calcium scanning in asymptomatic patients with diabetes mellitus: A paradigm shift. J Diab 2012;4:342–50.

is to start with CAC scanning. If any calcified plaque is detected, high risk has been established. If the CAC is 0, a low radiation dose (approximately 1 mSv) prospectively gated coronary CT angiography to evaluate for noncalcified plaque may be considered. With the progressive decrease in radiation dose, coronary CT angiography in patients as young as the 20s may be reasonable in selected cases. Repeat scanning in 4 to 5 years is appropriate if the initial test is entirely normal.

Young Patients

FH aside, the incidence of CAC greater than 0 in the 33- to 45-year age group is 9.9%; the percentages increase with increasing FRS (**Table 5**). Although CAC scanning is not guideline recommended in this age group, it can be helpful in decision making on starting statin usage in these younger individuals.

CORONARY ARTERY CALCIUM SCANNING AND ADHERENCE

Reviewing the CAC images with asymptomatic patients has consistently led to increased adherence to acetylsalicylic acid (aspirin) (ASA), statins, diet, and exercise (**Table 6**).[30–32]

Table 5
Yield of screening for CAC in middle-aged adults based on the 10-year FRS: the CARDIA study

FRS	>0 (%)	NNS	>100 (%)	NNS
Total	9.9		1.8	
0%–2.5%	7.3	14	1.3	79
2.6%–5%	20.2	5	2.4	41
5.1%–10%	19.1	5	3.5	29
>10%	44.8	2	17.2	6
>5%	22.7	3.6		
>2.5%	23.0	4.3		

Asymptomatic patients: 2831; 33–45 years.
Abbreviations: CARDIA, Coronary Artery Risk Development in Young Adults; NNS, number needed to scan.
Reproduced with permission of Wiley from Hecht HS, Narula J. Coronary artery calcium scanning in asymptomatic patients with diabetes mellitus: A paradigm shift. J Diab 2012;4:342–50.

In the Early Identification of Subclinical Atherosclerosis by Noninvasive Imaging Research (EISNER) trial, asymptomatic patients were randomized to using CAC to guide treatment or employing usual care.[33] CAC-directed care produced significant improvement in systolic blood pressure, low-density lipoprotein cholesterol (LDL-C), weight, and waist size compared with usual care, without an increase in downstream testing. Patients with CAC greater than 400 had greater improvement than those with 0 CAC (**Table 7**).

SERIAL CORONARY ARTERY CALCIUM SCANNING

After the initial CAC scan, repeat scanning may be used to determine the response to treatment. A significant increase in plaque burden, as opposed to not achieving a specific LDL-C goal, defines treatment failure. Without tracking subclinical atherosclerosis, the only method for assessing treatment failure is the occurrence of an event or the development of symptoms, at which point it may be too late. The ability to identify treatment nonresponders by progressive excessive increases in CAC offers the opportunity to intervene with more aggressive treatment and possibly affect outcomes. The validity of this reasoning depends on demonstrating adverse outcomes

Table 6
Effect of coronary calcium on patient adherence

Author	N	Follow-up (y)	CAC	Statin	ASA	Diet	Exercise	Statin + ASA
Kalia et al,[30] 2006	505	3.6	>400	90%				
			100–400	75%				
			1–99	63%				
			0	44%				
Orakzai et al,[31] 2008	980	3	>400			61%	67%	56%
			0			29%	33%	44%
Schmermund et al,[32] 2008	1640	6	>0 vs 0	OR 3.5	OR 3.1			OR 7.0

Abbreviation: OR, odds ratio.
Data from Refs.[30–32]

Table 7 EISNER trial			
Parameters	CACS = 0	CACS >400	P
Change in LDL-C	−12 mg/dL	−29 mg/dL	<.001
Change in SBP	−4 mm Hg	−9 mm Hg	<.001
Exercise	32%	47%	.03
New lipid Rx	19%	65%	<.001
New BP Rx	20%	46%	<.001
New ASA Rx	5%	21%	<.001
Lipid adherence	80%	88%	.04

Middle-aged patients (2137; 45–79 years) without CVD; 4-year follow-up; CAC treatment-directed versus usual care.
Abbreviations: BP, blood pressure; Rx, prescription; SBP, systolic blood pressure.
From Rozanski A, Gransar H, Shaw LJ, et al. Impact of coronary artery calcium scanning on coronary risk factors and downstream testing: the EISNER (Early Identification of Subclinical Atherosclerosis by Noninvasive Imaging Research) prospective randomized trial. J Am Coll Cardiol 2011;57:1627; with permission.

with plaque progression. Otherwise, calcification of preexisting noncalcified plaque could be invoked to explain an absence of increased risk. The data uniformly support the significant direct relationship between CAC progression and coronary events. In the Multi-Ethnic Study of Atherosclerosis (MESA), development of CAC in patients with 0 baseline scores and increases in CAC in those with greater than 0 baseline scores were associated with a poorer prognosis directly related to the extent of CAC progression (**Fig. 8**).[34] Although there is greater average CAC progression on statins versus no statins, those who start with a 0 CAC score and progress at a rate of 5 AU/year or those starting with a score greater than 0 AU and progress at a rate of greater than or equal to 15%/year have a 40% to 60% increase in event rates versus those who progress at lower rates over a 7.5-year follow-up.

The deleterious effects of CAC progression are more pronounced in patients with diabetes; similar progression yielded greater decreases in event-free survival in those with compared with those without diabetes (**Fig. 9**).[35]

The CAC progression-related risk is more pronounced in patients with diabetes and the metabolic syndrome compared with those with the metabolic syndrome alone (**Fig. 10**).[36]

Greater progression in patients on statins (see **Fig. 8**)[34] might have suggested greater conversion of noncalcified to calcified plaque by the drug, but greater progression in patients with events on statins negates this theory and implies a therapeutic failure of statins to sufficiently halt the atherosclerotic process. This emphasizes the fallacy in conventional thinking that statin treatment must slow progression because it is well known that "statins save lives." Statin monotherapy, however, produces no greater than a 44% event reduction compared with placebo,[37–40] and there are no data demonstrating differences in attained LDL-C between treated patients with and without events.

Inadequate treatment is demonstrated in **Fig. 11**, with excessive progression of CAC despite dramatic improvement in lipid values.

Even for patients on moderate or high statin doses, there is usually room for improvement, whether by further increases in LDL-C–lowering drugs, or intensifying lifestyle modification, the need for which can only be determined by repeat scanning.

6778 Patients, 45-84 years old
2 Scans: baseline and 2.5 years later
7.6-Year follow-up: 343 total, 206 hard events

Hazard Ratio		
0 Baseline CAC n = 3396		
Events	Total	Hard
Per 5 AU/y	1.4	1.5
>0 Baseline CAC n = 3382		
Per 100 AU/y	1.2	1.3
>300 AU/y	3.8	6.3
<5%/y	1.0	1.0
5%–14%/y	1.1	1.0
15%–29%/y	1.6	1.4
>30%/y	1.5	1.4

Progression (AU)	
No statins	46.2/y
Statins	60.0/y
P	<.001
Events	
No statins	55.7/y
Statins	119.3/y

Fig. 8. Coronary calcium progression and incident CHD events in MESA. (*Data from* Budoff MJ, Young R, Lopez VA. Progression of coronary calcium and incident coronary heart disease events: MESA [Multi-Ethnic Study of Atherosclerosis]. J Am Coll Cardiol 2013;61(12):1236, 1237.)

296 Asymptomatic patients with DM
300 Controls
59±6 years, 29% women
Scan interval 1–2 years
Follow-up 56±11 months

Event-Free Survival		
ΔCAC	DM	No DM
<10%	97.9%	100%
10%–20%	95.9%	97.2%
21%–30%	92.7%	94%
>30%	79.6%	90.6%

Death HR: DM vs Controls (N=596)			
ΔCAC	Matched Control Group	DM	P
10%–20% vs <10%	1.0	1.88	0.0001
21%–30% vs <10%	1.0	2.29	0.0001
>30% vs <10%	1.0	6.95	0.0001

*Adjusted for age, gender, HTN, HLP, FH of CHD, baseline CAC, and smoking

Fig. 9. Impact of CAC progression on outcome in subjects with and without diabetes. DM, diabetes mellitus; HLP, hyperlipidemia; HTN, hypertension. (*Data from* Kiramijyan S, Ahmadi N, Isma'eel H, et al. Impact of coronary artery calcium progression and statin therapy on clinical outcome in subjects with and without diabetes. Am J Cardiol 2013;111:358, 359.)

5662 Patients, 51% Female, 61.0 + 10.3 years, 4.9-year follow-up
2 Scans 2.4 years apart: 2927—0 baseline CAC
2735—>0 baseline CAC

RR for Events Related to CAC Progression			
	o Prog	2nd Tertile	3rd Tertile
+MetS/–DM	1	2.3	4.1
+MetS/+DM	1	4.1	8.5
P		<.05	<.05

Fig. 10. Metabolic syndrome, DM, and incidence and progression of CAC: MESA. DM, diabetes mellitus; MetS, metabolic syndrome. (Data from Wong ND, Nelson JC, Granston T, et al. Metabolic syndrome, diabetes, and incidence and progression of coro-nary calcium: the Multiethnic Study of Atherosclerosis [MESA]. JACC Cardiovasc Imaging 2012;5:363, 364.)

Continued progression in the setting of truly maximal treatment serves to identify patients who should be educated regarding the warning signs of acute coronary syndromes.

Asymptomatic patients with a 0 CAC score should not undergo repeat scanning for at least 4 years. The average time to conversion to a greater than 0 CAC was 4.1 ± 0.9 years and the average score at the time of conversion was 19 ± 19.[41]

The repeat scanning interval in patients with greater than 0 CAC is not data determined. Rather, logic dictates that the greater the concern, the shorter should be the interval. It seems reasonable to rescan after 2 years for CAC greater than 400 or greater than 75th percentile, with 3- or 4-year intervals for lower scores. The low radiation dose makes repeat scanning less problematic.

POST–CORONARY ARTERY CALCIUM SCANNING TESTING

The appropriateness of stress testing after CAC scanning in asymptomatic patients is directly related to the CAC score. The data indicate that the incidence of abnormal

43-year-old asymptomatic man, father, MI 41

Baseline: CAC 12

		Baseline	2 y
Lipids:	TC	244	163
	LDL	149	92
	HDL	39	52
	TG	280	94
Plaque:	Calcium score	12	56
	Calcium percentile	**75**	**89**
Treatment:	Statin	None	20 mg
	Niacin	None	2000 mg

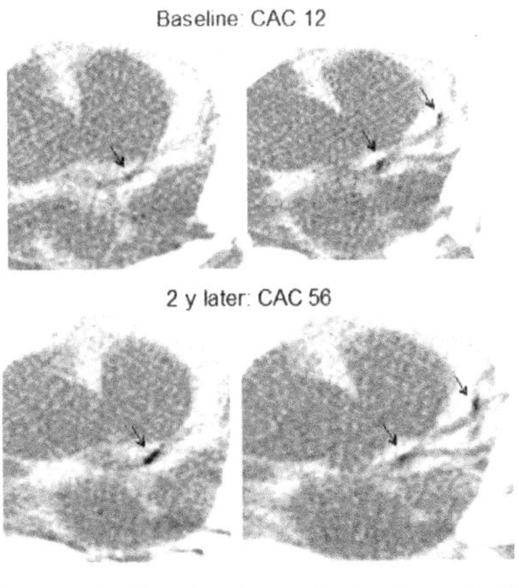

2 y later: CAC 56

Fig. 11. Progression of coronary artery calcium demonstrating inadequate treatment. MI, myocardial infarction.

nuclear stress testing is 1.3%, 11.3%, and 35.2% for CAC scores of less than 100, 100 to 400, and greater than 400, respectively.[42–46] It is only in the greater than 400 group that the pretest likelihood is sufficiently high to warrant further evaluation with functional testing. Coronary CT angiography is appropriate in patients with CAC less than 1000; higher CAC scores may preclude accurate evaluation. It is never appropriate to proceed directly to the catheterization laboratory in asymptomatic patients.

Evaluation of incidental findings, in particular lung nodules, should follow standard radiology guidelines.[47]

CORONARY ARTERY CALCIUM SCANNING AND THE 2013 GUIDELINES

The 2010 ACCF/AHA Guideline for Assessment of Cardiovascular Risk in Asymptomatic Adults appropriately assigned a class IIa recommendation to CAC for evaluation of the asymptomatic intermediate-risk population and for all patients older than 40 with diabetes mellitus.[21] The 2013 American College of Cardiology (ACC)/AHA Guideline on the Treatment of Blood Cholesterol to Reduce Atherosclerotic Cardiovascular Risk in Adults[48] and the 2013 ACC/AHA Guideline on the Assessment of Cardiovascular Risk[49] have reversed course and downgraded CAC to a class IIb recommendation. Assuming that the goal of guidelines is to use the most powerful predictors of risk to direct treatment, it is difficult to understand how the most powerful risk predictor (ie, CAC) has been downgraded from earlier documents rather than further upgraded based on robust data published after the 2010 ACCF/AHA guideline.[21] The explanations for the downgrading of CAC to class IIb can only be understood as follows:

1. The outcomes on which the 2013 guidelines were based were changed by the addition of stroke, for which the investigators believed there was not sufficient CAC data, even though the Heinz Nixdorf Recall Study of 4180 patients demonstrated hazard ratios of CAC for stroke to be similar to age, hypertension, and smoking (**Table 8**).[50]

Consequently, the CAC data for coronary risk was essentially discarded and the recommendation lowered to IIb.

Table 8
Coronary artery calcium is an independent predictor of stroke in the general population: the Heinz Nixdorf Recall Study

	CAC	
	CVA	**No CVA**
Median	104.8	11.2
Q1;Q3	14.0;482.2	0;106.2
P		<.001
	Hazard Ratio	**P**
log10 (CAC + 1)	1.52	.001
Age/5 y	1.35	<.001
SBP/10 mm	1.25	<.001
Smoking	1.75	.025

Patients: 4180; 45–75 years; 47.1% men; 94.9 ± 19–month follow-up.
Data from Hermann DM, Gronewold J, Lehmann N, et al, Heinz Nixdorf Recall Study Investigative Group. Coronary artery calcification is an independent stroke predictor in the general population. Stroke 2013;44:1008–13.

2. Erroneous cost and radiation exposure concerns were also invoked to justify the IIb classification. In reality, the cost of CAC scanning has dramatically decreased to the approximately $100 level, and a recent analysis demonstrated that treating 7.5% 10-year risk patients with statins at a $1/pill cost who had CAC greater than 0 resulted in cost per quality-adjusted life year saved of $18,000 compared with $78,000 for risk factor assessment alone.[51] The radiation issue has become less relevant as the dosage has progressively decreased to 1 mSv or less.

3. The guidelines noted that the class IIb recommendation is consistent with the recommendations in the 2010 ACCF/AHA guideline for patients with a 10-year coronary heart disease (CHD); risk of less than 10%.[21] It is totally inconsistent, however, with the class IIa 2010 guideline recommendation for the 10% to 20% group,[21] which is now excluded from CAC evaluation because they will all receive statins by the new recommendations. It is precisely this large group for which the NRI by CAC in 3 major population-based prospective outcome studies[11,15,16] has ranged from 52% to 66% (see **Table 3**). Moreover, as demonstrated in every outcome study comparing CAC to conventional risk factor–based assessment, CAC is superior to risk factors.

4. The most persistent criticism of CAC has been the absence of randomized controlled trials (RCTs) that demonstrate its ability to improve outcomes. The 2013 guidelines acknowledge, however, that their new risk assessment paradigm has also not been formally evaluated in randomized controlled trials.

In summary, the 2013 guidelines, under the mantle of dedication to RCTs, have presented a non–RCT-validated risk assessment paradigm, which is erroneous in at least 50% of the 7.5% to 20% 10-year risk group, and have downgraded CAC to a IIb recommendation for whom only those few patients who are not in their 4 primary risk categories will be eligible. Consequently, with respect to CAC, the 2010 guideline, rather than the 2013 guidelines, should be implemented.

CORONARY ARTERY CALCIUM SCANNING LIMITATIONS

1. CAC is not a perfect test and events do occur in the setting of a 0 CAC. Only 5% of acute myocardial infarctions or unstable angina occur, however, in both younger (mean age 47 years) and older (mean age 57 years) patients with a 0 CAC (**Fig. 12**).[52,53]
   In asymptomatic patients with 0 CAC, the incidence of obstructive CAD is less than 1%; in patients with chest pain and 0 CAC, it is approximately 5%.

2. Radiation is no longer a significant issue because the absorbed radiation dose falls to the level of mammography. Unfortunately, irresponsible scare tactics have magnified public concern; education is needed to counter these negative effects.

3. Cost has also become less of a concern as the price of CAC scanning has plummeted to approximately $100. As discussed previously, cost-effectiveness analyses highly favor CAC.

4. Incidentalomas and their subsequent evaluation have generated negative sentiments. The frequency of clinically significant findings is 1.2%, with indeterminate findings at 7.0%.[54] The associated costs do not have a negative impact on the cost effectiveness of CAC.[51] Standard guidelines on how to handle these findings may reassure patients and physicians.[47]

5. Patient anxiety related to CAC findings has also been cited as a negative. Anxiety is not an intended consequence but a certain amount is appropriate and inevitable

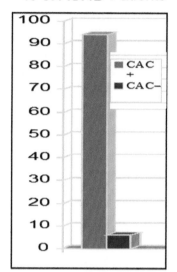

114 Patients: MI (97) or UA (17)
Age: 57 ± 11 y

% of ASHD Patients

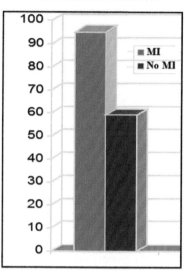

102 Patients < 60 with MI
Age: 41 ± 7 y

Calcium Present

Fig. 12. Coronary calcium in patients with first myocardial infarction (MI) or unstable angina (UA). (*Data from* Schmermund A, Baumgart D, Görge G, et al. Coronary artery calcium in acute coronary syndromes: a comparative study of electron-beam computed tomography, coronary angiography, and intracoronary ultrasound in survivors of acute myocardial infarction and unstable angina. Circulation 1997;96:1465, with permission; and Pohle K, Ropers D, Mäffert R, et al. Coronary calcifications in young patients with first, unheralded myocardial infarction: a risk factor matched analysis by electron beam tomography. Heart 2003;89:627.)

when informed of increased cardiac risk and may motivate increased adherence. On the other hand, for those with high anxiety of early arteriosclerotic cardiovascular disease (ASCVD) based on a severe FH or a high calculated ASCVD risk score, concern can often be calmed when reclassified toward significantly less risk by CAC.

SUMMARY

The potential impact of CAC on primary prevention cannot be overestimated. It eliminates the guesswork implicit in extrapolating risk from guidelines derived from large population bases to individual patients and provides a snapshot of the cumulative effect of an individual's life on the coronary circulation. The role of risk factors is most important in identifying treatable therapeutic targets after risk has been established by a test that is 100% specific for atherosclerosis and far superior to any risk factor–based paradigm. The remaining barriers include physician education to overcome instinctive clinging to the old established paradigms, patient education to increase awareness of the widespread availability and low radiation of CAC, and more widespread insurance reimbursement.

REFERENCES

1. Canto JG, Kiefe CI, Rogers WJ, et al. Number of coronary heart disease risk factors and mortality in patients with first myocardial infarction. JAMA 2011;306: 2120–7.
2. Arad Y, Spadaro LA, Goodman K, et al. Prediction of coronary events with electron beam computed tomography. J Am Coll Cardiol 2000;36:1253–60.
3. Park R, Robert Detrano R, Xiang M, et al. Combined use of computed tomography coronary calcium scores and C-reactive protein levels in predicting cardiovascular events in nondiabetic individuals. Circulation 2002;106:2073–7.
4. Raggi P, Callister TQ, Cooil B, et al. Identification of patients at increased risk of first unheralded acute myocardial infarction by electron beam computed tomography. Circulation 2000;101:850–5.
5. Wong ND, Hsu JC, Detrano RC, et al. Coronary artery calcium evaluation by electron beam compute tomography and its relation to new cardiovascular events. Am J Cardiol 2000;86:495–8.
6. Kondos GT, Hoff JA, Sevrukov A, et al. Electron-beam tomography coronary artery calcium and cardiac events: a 37-month follow-up of 5,635 initially asymptomatic low to intermediate risk adults. Circulation 2003;107:2571–6.
7. Greenland P, LaBree L, Azen SP, et al. Coronary artery calcium score combined with Framingham score for risk prediction in asymptomatic individuals. JAMA 2004;291:10.
8. Shaw LJ, Raggi P, Schisterman E, et al. Prognostic value of cardiac risk factors and coronary artery calcium screening for all- cause mortality. Radiology 2003; 28:826–33.
9. Arad Y, Goodman KJ, Roth M, et al. Coronary calcification, coronary risk factors, and atherosclerotic cardiovascular disease events. The St Francis Heart Study. J Am Coll Cardiol 2005;46(1):158–65.
10. Taylor AJ, Bindeman J, Feuerstein I, et al. Coronary calcium independently predicts incident premature coronary heart disease over measured cardiovascular risk factors mean three-year out- comes in the Prospective Army Coronary Calcium (PACC) project. J Am Coll Cardiol 2005;46:807–14.
11. Vliegenthart R, Oudkerk M, Song B, et al. Coronary calcification detected by electron-beam computed tomography and myocardial infarction. The Rotterdam Coronary Calcification Study. Eur Heart J 2002;23:1596–603.
12. Budoff MJ, Shaw LJ, Liu ST, et al. Long-term prognosis associated with coronary calcification. Observations from a registry of 25, 253 patients. J Am Coll Cardiol 2007;49:1860–70.
13. Lakoski SG, Greenland P, Wong ND, et al. Coronary artery calcium scores and risk for cardiovascular events in women classified as "Low Risk" based on Framingham risk score. The Multi-Ethnic Study of Atherosclerosis (MESA). Arch Intern Med 2007;167(22):2437–42.
14. Becker A, Leber A, Becker C, et al. Predictive value of coronary calcifications for future cardiac events in asymptomatic individuals. Am Heart J 2008;155: 154–60.
15. Detrano R, Guerci AD, Carr JJ, et al. Coronary calcium as a predictor of coronary events in four racial or ethnic groups. N Engl J Med 2008;358:1336–45.
16. Erbel R, Möhlenkamp S, Moebus S, et al. Coronary risk stratification, discrimination, and reclassification improvement based on quantification of subclinical coronary atherosclerosis. The Heinz Nixdorf Recall Study. J Am Coll Cardiol 2010;56:1397–406.

17. Taylor AJ, Fiorillia PN, Hongyan W, et al. Relation between the Framingham risk score, coronary calcium, and incident coronary heart disease among low-risk men. Am J Cardiol 2010;106:47–50.
18. Nasir K, Rubin J, Blaha MJ, et al. Interplay of coronary artery calcification and traditional risk factors for the prediction of all-cause mortality in asymptomatic individuals. Circ Cardiovasc Imaging 2012;5:467–73.
19. Yeboah J, McClelland RL, Polonsky TS, et al. Comparison of novel risk markers for improvement in cardiovascular risk assessment in intermediate-risk individuals. JAMA 2012;308:788–95.
20. Rana JS, Gransar H, Wong ND, et al. Comparative value of coronary artery calcium and multiple blood biomarkers for prognostication of cardiovascular events. Am J Cardiol 2012;109:1449–53.
21. Greenland P, Alpert JS, Beller GA, et al. 2010 ACCF/AHA Guideline for assessment of cardiovascular risk in adults. A report of the American College of Cardiology Foundation/American Heart Association Task Force on Practice Guidelines. J Am Coll Cardiol 2010;56:e50–103.
22. Wong ND, Sciammarella MG, Polk D, et al. The metabolic syndrome, diabetes, and subclinical atherosclerosis assessed by coronary calcium. J Am Coll Cardiol 2003;41:1547–53.
23. Becker A, Leber A, Becker B, et al. Predictive value of coronary calcifications for future cardiac events in asymptomatic patients with diabetes mellitus: prospective study in 716 patients over 8 years. BMC Cardiovasc Disord 2008;27:1–8.
24. Elkeles R, Godsland IF, Feher MD, et al. Coronary cal- cium measurement improves prediction of cardiovascular events in asymptomatic patients with type 2 diabetes: the PREDICT study. Eur Heart J 2008;29:2244–51.
25. Anand DV, Lim E, Hopkins D, et al. Risk stratification in uncomplicated type 2 diabetes: prospective evaluation of the combined use of coronary artery calcium imaging and selective myocardial perfusion scintigraphy. Eur Heart J 2006;27:713–21.
26. Malik S, Budoff M, Katz R. Impact of subclinical atherosclerosis on cardiovascular disease events in individuals with metabolic syndrome and diabetes: the multi-ethnic study of atherosclerosis. Diabetes Care 2011;34:2285–90.
27. Kashani M, Eliasson A, Vernalis M, et al. Improving assessment of cardiovascular disease risk by using family history. J Cardiovasc Nurs 2013;28:E18–27.
28. Taylor A, Cerqueira M, Hodgson JM, et al. Appropriate use criteria for cardiac computed tomography. J Am Coll Cardiol 2010;56:1864–94.
29. Okwuosa TM, Greenland P, Burke GL, et al. Prediction of coronary artery calcium progression in individuals with low Framingham risk score: the multi-ethnic study of atherosclerosis. JACC Cardiovasc Imaging 2012;5:923–30.
30. Kalia NK, Miller LG, Nasir K, et al. Visualizing coronary calcium is associated with improvements in adherence to statin therapy. Atherosclerosis 2006;185:394–9.
31. Orakzai RH, Nasir K, Orakzai SH, et al. Effect of patient visualization of coronary calcium by electron beam computed tomography on changes in beneficial lifestyle behaviors. Am J Cardiol 2008;101:999–1002.
32. Schmermund A, Baumgart A, Taylor AJ, et al. Community-based provision of statin and aspirin after the detection of coronary artery calcium within a community-based screening cohort. J Am Coll Cardiol 2008;51:1337–41.
33. Rozanski A, Gransar H, Shaw LJ, et al. Impact of coronary artery calcium scanning on coronary risk factors and downstream testing: the EISNER (Early Identification of Subclinical Atherosclerosis by Noninvasive Imaging Research) prospective randomized trial. J Am Coll Cardiol 2011;57:1622–32.

34. Budoff MJ, Young R, Lopez VA, et al. Progression of coronary calcium and incident coronary heart disease events: MESA (Multi-Ethnic Study of Atherosclerosis). J Am Coll Cardiol 2013;61:1231–9.

35. Kiramijyan S, Ahmadi N, Isma'eel H, et al. Impact of coronary artery calcium progression and statin therapy on clinical outcome in subjects with and without diabetes. Am J Cardiol 2013;111:356–61.

36. Wong ND, Nelson JC, Granston T, et al. Metabolic syndrome, diabetes, and incidence and progression of coro- nary calcium: the Multiethnic Study of Atherosclerosis (MESA). JACC Cardiovasc Imaging 2012;5:358–66.

37. Scandinavian Simvastatin Survival Study Group. Randomised trial of cholesterol lowering in 4444 patients with coronary heart disease: the Scandinavian SimvastatinSurvival Study (4S). Lancet 1994;344:1383–9.

38. Sacks FM, Moyé LA, Davis BR, et al. Relationship between plasma LDL concentrations during treatment with pravastatin and recurrent coronary events in the cholesterol and recurrent events trial. Circulation 1998;97: 1446–52.

39. Prevention of cardiovascular events and death with pravastatin in patients with coronary heart disease and a broad range of initial cholesterol levels. The Long-Term Intervention with Pravastatin in Ischaemic Disease (LIPID) study group. N Engl J Med 1998;339:1349–57.

40. Ridker PM, Danielson E, Fonseca FA, et al. Rosuvastatin to prevent vascular events in men and women with elevated C-reactive protein. N Engl J Med 2008;359:2195–207.

41. Min JK, Lin FY, Gidseg DS, et al. Determinants of coronary calcium conversion among patients with a normal coronary calcium scan. What is the "warranty period" for remaining normal? J Am Coll Cardiol 2010;55:1110–7.

42. He ZX, Hedrick TD, Pratt CM, et al. Severity of coronary artery calcification by electron beam computed tomography predicts silent myocardial ischemia. Circulation 2000;101:244–51.

43. Moser KW, O'Keefe JH, Bateman TM, et al. Coronary calcium screening in asymptomatic patients as a guide to risk factor modification and stress myocardial perfusion imaging. J Nucl Cardiol 2003;10:590–8.

44. Berman DS, Wong ND, Gransar H, et al. Relationship between stress-induced myocardial ischemia and atherosclerosis measured by coronary calcium tomography. J Am Coll Cardiol 2004;44:923–30.

45. Anand DJ, Lim E, Raval U, et al. Prevalence of silent myocardial ischemia in asymptomatic individuals with subclinical atherosclerosis detected by electron beam tomography. J Nucl Cardiol 2004;11:450–7.

46. Su Min Chang SM, Faisal Nabi F, Xu J, et al. The coronary artery calcium score and stress myocardial perfusion imaging provide independent and complementary prediction of cardiac risk. J Am Coll Cardiol 2009;54: 1872–82.

47. MacMahon H, Austin JH, Gamsu G, et al. Guidelines for management of small pulmonary nodules detected on CT scans: a statement from the Fleischner Society. Radiology 2005;237:395–400.

48. Stone NJ, Robinson J, Lichtenstein AH, et al. 2013 ACC/AHA guideline on the treatment of blood cholesterol to reduce atherosclerotic cardiovascular risk in adults. J Am Coll Cardiol 2013. http://dx.doi.org/10.1016/j.jacc.2013.11.002.

49. Goff DC Jr, Lloyd-Jones DM, Bennett G, et al. 2013 ACC/AHA guideline on the assessment of cardiovascular risk. J Am Coll Cardiol 2013. http://dx.doi.org/10.1016/j.jacc.2013.11.005.

50. Hermann DM, Gronewold J, Lehmann N, et al. Coronary artery calcification is an independent stroke predictor in the general population. Stroke 2013;44: 1008–13.
51. Pletcher MJ, Pignone M, Earnshaw S, et al. Using the coronary artery calcium score to guide statin therapy. A cost-effectiveness analysis. Circ Cardiovasc Qual Outcomes 2014;7:276–84.
52. Schmermund A, Baumgart D, Görge G, et al. Coronary artery calcium in acute coronary syndromes: a comparative study of electron-beam computed tomography, coronary angiography, and intracoronary ultrasound in survivors of acute myocardial infarction and unstable angina. Circulation 1997;96:1461–9.
53. Pohle K, Ropers D, Mäffert R, et al. Coronary calcifications in young patients with first, unheralded myocardial infarction: a risk factor matched analysis by electron beam tomography. Heart 2003;89:625–8.
54. MacHaalany J, Yeung Y, Ruddy TD, et al. Potential clinical and economic consequences of noncardiac incidental findings on cardiac computed tomography. J Am Coll Cardiol 2009;54:1533–4.

Beginning to Understand High-Density Lipoproteins

Carlos G. Santos-Gallego, MD, Juan J. Badimon, PhD, Robert S. Rosenson, MD*

KEYWORDS

- High-density lipoprotein • Apolipoprotein A-I • High-density lipoprotein particles
- Reverse cholesterol transport • Atherosclerosis • Niacin • Fibrates
- Cholesteryl ester transfer protein inhibitor

KEY POINTS

- High-density lipoprotein (HDL) cholesterol (HDL-C) has been considered to reduce the risk for atherosclerotic cardiovascular disease (CVD).
- Contradictory evidence has appeared in the last years, including the lack of inverse association between HDL-C and CVD risk in the presence of very low levels of low-density lipoprotein cholesterol (LDL-C), and the failure of novel pharmacologic strategies targeting increases in HDL-C.
- Cholesterol implicated in the reverse cholesterol transport contributes only 5% of all the clinically measured HDL-C; therefore, HDL-C levels (or the change in them) are not a precise parameter for adequately assessment of the contribution of HDL to CVD risk.
- The cholesterol content of HDL does not represent many important HDL functions that are related to CVD risk, such as antioxidant, anti-inflammatory, antiapoptotic, and vasorelaxant properties. Therefore, a need exists to move beyond HDL-C as a surrogate for the beneficial actions of HDL.
- HDL particle concentration is a better biomarker than HDL-C, because it predicts CVD risk even after adjusting for HDL-C and also in the presence of very low levels of LDL-C.

INTRODUCTION

For the last 60 years, high-density lipoproteins (HDL) have been widely considered to reduce the risk for cardiovascular disease (CVD); in fact, the cholesterol carried by HDL (HDL-C) has earned the moniker of "good cholesterol". This concept has led to the development of several pharmacologic strategies aiming to raise HDL-C to reduce

Disclosures: None (C.G. Santos-Gallego, J.J. Badimon); Grant/Research Support: AstraZeneca, Amgen, Hoffman-LaRoche, Sanofi; Consultant/Advisor: Aegerion, Amgen, Astra Zeneca, Eli Lilly, Janssen, LipoScience, Novartis, Regeneron, Sanofi; Equity Interests/Stock Options: LipoScience, (R.S. Rosenson).
Cardiovascular Institute, Icahn School of Medicine at Mount Sinai, One Gustave Levy Place, Box 1030, New York, NY 10029, USA
* Corresponding author.
E-mail address: robert.rosenson@mssm.edu

Endocrinol Metab Clin N Am 43 (2014) 913–947
http://dx.doi.org/10.1016/j.ecl.2014.08.001
0889-8529/14/$ – see front matter © 2014 Elsevier Inc. All rights reserved.

endo.theclinics.com

CVD risk. The proposition that HDL protects against the development of cardiovascular diseases is based on several robust and consistent observations: (1) numerous human population studies have shown that the plasma concentrations of both HDL-C and the major HDL apolipoprotein (apo), apoA-I, are independent, inverse predictors of the risk of having a CVD event (**Table 1**). Moreover, low HDL-C remains predictive of increased CVD, even when low-density lipoprotein (LDL) cholesterol (LDL-C) has been reduced to low levels by treatment with statins[1]; (2) HDL have several well-documented functions with the potential to protect against cardiovascular disease (see later discussion); (3) interventions that increase the concentration of HDL inhibit the development and progression of atherosclerosis in several animal models[2–4]; and (4) in proof-of-concept studies in humans, intravenous infusions of reconstituted HDL (rHDL) consisting of apoA-I complexed with phospholipids promote regression of coronary atheroma as assessed by intravascular ultrasonography.[5,6]

However, the hypothesis that HDL-C and apoA-I directly confer biological protection against atherosclerosis has never been proved. The same is true for the hypothesis that raising HDL-C or apoA-I levels will result in reduced CVD risk. In fact, several recent lines of evidence have questioned HDL-C and apoA-I as relevant therapeutic targets. First, a recent study showed that some genetic variants that raise HDL-C levels are not associated with a proportionally lower risk of myocardial infarction.[7] Second, a subanalysis of the JUPITER trial has shown that HDL-C and apoA-I were associated with reduced CVD risk among patients in the placebo arm, but that this association was lost among people on rosuvastatin 20 mg achieving very low levels of LDL-C.[8] Third, data from population studies and from a meta-analysis have suggested that changes in HDL-C levels after initiation of lipid-modifying therapy are not independently associated with CVD risk.[9,10] Finally, recent clinical trials have shown that HDL-C–raising pharmacologic therapy increases HDL-C levels but does not reduce CVD events (eg, AIM-HIGH[11] and HPS-THRIVE[12] for niacin, dal-OUTCOMES[13] for dalcetrapib, ACCORD[14] for fenofibrate).

This review attempts to reconcile the beneficial effects of HDL metabolism on CVD risk with the more recent studies, which seem to cast a shadow on the future of HDL by formulating a comprehensive hypothesis that includes both facts. Finally, current and future pharmacologic strategies targeting HDL are discussed.

COMPOSITION OF THE HIGH-DENSITY LIPOPROTEIN PARTICLES

A crucial distinction must be made between HDL-C (ie, the amount of cholesterol carried by the HDL) and the HDL particle (HDL-P, the individual molecule containing proteins and lipids—specifically cholesterol but also other types of lipids). The levels of HDL-C do not necessarily reflect the concentration of HDL-P because HDL-P can be fully or only partially loaded with cholesterol. This distinction is key to shedding light on the recent seeming "failings" of the protective role of HDL-C in CVD.

HDL-P is a complex and heterogeneous assembly of proteins, lipids, and microRNAs (miRNA).

- *Proteome composition of HDL-P.* Approximately 75% of the protein content of HDL is apoA-I, which serves as the primary protein scaffolding on which the lipid cargo-carrying particle is built. Each HDL particle contains 2 to 5 molecules of apoA-I,[15,16] so apoA-I levels provide no indication of the HDL-P concentration. Other protein components of HDL are apoA-II, apoA-IV, apoA-V, apoE, apoJ, apoM, lecithin-cholesterol acyl transferase (LCAT), cholesteryl ester transfer protein (CETP), and the antioxidant enzymes paroxonase 1 (PON-1) and glutathione selenoperoxidase.

Table 1
Epidemiologic studies suggesting an inverse relationship between HDL-C concentrations and CVD risk

Study	Population	Methods	Results
Tromsø Heart Study[179]	6595 males, age 20–49 y	Population screening, followed for 2 y	HDL-C level was inversely correlated with CV risk. HDL-C was 3 times better than non–HDL-C for CVD risk prediction
Framingham Heart Study[180]	1605 patients, age 49–82 y	16 groups stratified by HDL and TC levels, followed for 12 y	High levels of HDL-C were shown to correlate with lower incidences of CHD for all levels of TC (1 mg/dL increase in HDL correlated with 2%–3% decrease in CHD risk)
MRFIT (Multiple Risk Factor – Intervention Trial)[181]	5792 males with elevated CHD risk factors, age 35–57 y	Risk factor modification vs no intervention, followed for 7 y	No change in HDL levels; no significant difference in CHD mortality
Lipid Research Clinics Coronary Primary Prevention Trial[182]	1808 males with hyperlipidemia, age 30–69 y	Lipid-lowering diet + placebo vs cholestyramine, followed for 7 y	In both the drug and placebo groups, a 1 mg/dL increase in HDL was associated with a 3.4%–5.5% reduction in primary CHD events
Prospective Cardiovascular Munster (PROCAM)[183]	19,698 volunteers (4559 males between 40 and 64 y were analyzed)	Followed for 6 y	Subjects with HDL <35 mg/dL showed 4 times greater CV risk
Israeli Ischemic Heart Disease Study (Gouldbort)[184]	8565 males, age >42 y	4 groups stratified by HDL and TC levels, followed for 21 y	Subgroups with low HDL-C had a 35% higher CV mortality rate than those groups with high HDL-C (even after adjusting by age and other CV risk factors)
Atherosclerosis Risk in Communities (ARIC) Study[185]	12,339 participants, age 45–64 y	Followed for 10 y	Inverse relation between HDL-C and CV risk. Risk prediction by HDL-C seems to be greater in females than in males
Prospective Epidemiological Study of Myocardial Infarction (PRIME)[186]	10,592 volunteers, age 50–59 y	Prospective cohort study, followed for 5 y	A significant (P<.0001) linear increase in relative CVD risk was observed for HDL-C decrease. The levels of apoA-I were also predictive.

Abbreviations: ApoA-I, apolipoprotein A-I; CHD, coronary heart disease; CV, cardiovascular; CVD, cardiovascular disease; TC, total cholesterol.
Data from Refs.[179–186]

- *Lipidome composition of the HDL-P.* The lipid composition of HDL-P is also rich, because it mainly contains cholesteryl esters (CE) but also other lipids such as free cholesterol (FC), triglycerides (TG), and phospholipids (PL). PL and FC form the surface lipid monolayer of HDL-P, while CE and TG build the hydrophobic lipid core. Of interesting, PL quantitatively predominate in the HDL lipidome (accounting for 20%–30% of total HDL mass), followed by CE (14%–18%), TG (3%–6%), and FC (3%–5%).[17] The lysophospholipid sphingosine-1-phosphate (S1P) is also predominantly carried by the HDL-P, and has recently been demonstrated to specifically possess antiatherosclerotic effects.[18–20]

- *micro RNA (miRNA)* are small (~22 nucleotides), noncoding RNA, which bind to partially complementary sites primarily found in the 3'-untranslated region of target mRNAs and which inhibit gene expression via induction of mRNA degradation. Although miRNAs act intracellularly, they can be exported in exosomes and microparticles. Recently, HDL-P have been discovered to transport miRNA,[21] and HDL-P are much more enriched in miRNA than LDL particles (LDL-P). Furthermore, HDL-mediated delivery of miRNAs to recipient cells was demonstrated to be dependent on scavenger receptor class B type I (SR-BI).[21] Moreover, HDL-P are much more enriched than LDL-P in miRNA,[22] and miR-223, miR-126, and miR-92 are detected with the higher number of copies.[22] Preliminary reports suggested that the human HDL-miRNA profile of normal subjects is significantly different from that of CVD patients,[21] but data seem contradictory.[22]

Molar differences in the content of major proteins and lipid constituents of HDL cause considerable heterogeneity of HDL as delineated by electron microscopy (shape), ultracentrifugation (density), gel filtration, polyacrylamide gel electrophoresis, nuclear magnetic resonance spectroscopy (size), charge (agarose gel electrophoresis), or affinity (apolipoprotein composition); unfortunately, there is overlap between the proposed HDL subclasses defined by the various isolation methods. To homogenize the concepts and facilitate communication, the authors have previously proposed a uniform standardized nomenclature[23] of 5 HDL subclasses according to size that allows clinicians and scientists to be consistent in their definitions.

OVERVIEW OF HIGH-DENSITY LIPOPROTEIN METABOLIC PATHWAYS: REVERSE CHOLESTEROL TRANSPORT

The purpose of this review is to propose an explanation about the discordant later results with HDL as a therapeutic target. Therefore, the metabolism of HDL is only succinctly summarized (**Fig. 1**; for a more detailed explanation, see Refs.[24–26]).

In contrast to LDL, HDL requires a maturation process. ApoA-I is expressed and secreted predominantly by the liver (70%) and also by the small intestine (30%). Lipid-free apoA-I rapidly obtains small amounts of PL[25] (very small HDL [HDL-VS] in the standardized nomenclature, also called pre-β migrating HDL). These HDL-VS bind to adenosine triphosphate (ATP)-binding cassette transporter A1 (ABCA1) on liver, intestine, or macrophages, thus acquiring FC, increasing its lipid content and becoming discoid-shaped larger HDL particles (small HDL [HDL-S]).

LCAT catalyzes the transfer of an acyl group from lecithin to FC and generates hydrophobic CE, which migrate to the core of HDL-P thus leading to the formation of spherical mature particles (medium HDL [HDL-M] in the standardized nomenclature). Mature HDL-M bind with receptors ATP-binding cassette transporter G1 (ABCG1) and SR-BI, which are responsible for additional cholesterol efflux to mature HDL particles, further increasing the size and CE content of the now buoyant and

Increase Preβ-HDL and ApoA-I

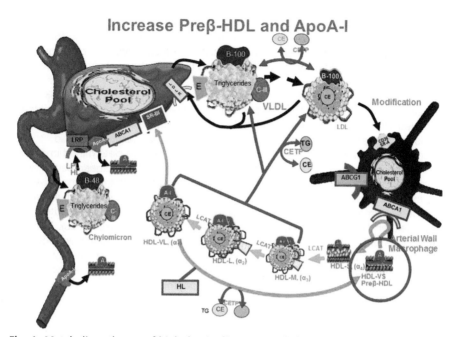

Fig. 1. Metabolic pathways of high-density lipoprotein cholesterol and reverse cholesterol transport in humans. ABCA1, adenosine triphosphate (ATP)-binding cassette transporter A1; ABCG1, ATP-binding cassette transporter G1; Apo, apolipoprotein; CE, cholesteryl ester; CETP, cholesteryl ester transfer protein; HDL, high-density lipoprotein (-VS, very small; -S, small; -M, medium; -L, large; -VL, very large); HL, hepatic lipase; LCAT, lecithin-cholesterol acyl transferase; LDLR, low-density lipoprotein receptor; LPL, lipoprotein lipase; LRP, lipoprotein receptor–related protein; TG, triglycerides; VLDL, very low-density lipoprotein. (*Courtesy of* H. Bryan Brewer Jr, MD, Washington, DC, and Robert S. Rosenson, MD, New York, NY.)

spherical HDL particle (large HDL [HDL-L] and very large HDL [HDL-VL] in the standardized nomenclature).

The reverse cholesterol transport (RCT) loop is closed with CE delivery to the liver by 2 different mechanisms. First, HDL-L and HDL-VL are selectively taken up in the liver by means of hepatic SR-BI receptors, thus completing cholesterol return to the liver. In addition, CETP transfers CE from HDL particles to TG-rich lipoproteins (very low-density lipoprotein [VLDL] and LDL); cholesterol finally reaches the liver when LDL-P are taken up by the liver via the LDL receptor.

There is functional heterogeneity among the different HDL particles. HDL-S and HDL-VS particles are most efficient in interacting with the ABCA1 to promote cholesterol efflux from cells, whereas HDL-L and HDL-VL are the most efficient in interacting with liver SR-BI for delivery of cholesterol to the liver.[23] HDL-M particles are the ones most interactive with ABCG1 to promote cellular cholesterol efflux.[23] Specifically, HDL-VS seem to be very active; in fact, delipidated HDL or apoA-I Milano complexed with phospholipids (which can be assimilated to HDL-VS) have been shown to promote regression of coronary atherosclerosis.[5,6] Therefore, because some HDL-P are more effective than others at cholesterol efflux, the number and size of the HDL-P (ie, the capacity to accept more cholesterol) seems to be much more relevant for HDL antiatherosclerotic effects than the absolute concentration of HDL-C.

Only 3% to 5% of the mass of HDL-P, however, is derived from macrophage cholesterol efflux.[25] Thus, the fraction of cholesterol in HDL-P specifically corresponding to macrophage cholesterol efflux (ie, responsible for the antiatherosclerotic effect of HDL) is very small and most likely does not change HDL-C levels.[25] Therefore, HDL-C concentrations may be either an insensitive or ineffective method to quantify cholesterol changes in the vascular macrophages that have been proposed to reduce CVD events.

However, the use of multiple static measures of the pool size of HDL-C is likely an inadequate approach for the characterization of a dynamic process such as the afore-mentioned RCT and HDL metabolism. For these reasons, different experimental models for assessing the dynamic macrophage RCT have been developed.[25,27] At present, in vivo quantification of macrophage RCT can only be determined in animal models (murine model of intraperitoneal injection of macrophages loaded with tritium-labeled cholesterol) or through kinetic modeling of isotope dilution.[25,27] Clinically, ex vivo assays have been used to assess the capacity of individual patient serum and HDL specimens to remove cholesterol from cultured cholesterol-loaded macrophages (either J774 mouse macrophages or THP-1 human macrophages). Relative contributions of the efflux pathways in murine macrophages are as follows: ABCA1, 35%; aqueous diffusion, 35%; ABCG1, 21%; and SR-BI, 9%. In cholesterol-loaded human macrophages, the relative contributions of these pathways to cholesterol efflux are different; the ABCA1 pathway remains predominant, but ABCG1 does not contribute to efflux, and the SR-BI pathway is relatively more important.[25] A recent study reported that the capacity of individual patient serum to stimulate cholesterol efflux from J774 macrophages has a strong inverse association with angiographically quantified coronary artery disease (CAD) that was statistically independent of HDL-C or apoA-I levels.[28,29] Regarding carotid territories, cholesterol efflux capacity is also inversely associated with carotid intima-media thickness (cIMT),[28] with increasing carotid stenosis[30] and with more advanced carotid plaque morphology.[30] This result confirms that the functionality of HDL-P (determined by the size and concentration of HDL-P), but not the levels of HDL-C, is the main determinant of the beneficial effect of HDL. Surprisingly, some investigators have reported that an increased cholesterol efflux was paradoxically associated with a higher rate of CVD events[29]; however, one should consider that the overall number of events was low, and the definitive answer to the relationship of cholesterol efflux capacity to CVD events awaits much larger prospective cohort analyses.

ATHEROPROTECTIVE EFFECTS OF HIGH-DENSITY LIPOPROTEIN CHOLESTEROL INDEPENDENT OF REVERSE CHOLESTEROL TRANSPORT

Besides its cholesterol efflux capacity, HDL is well known to possess additional salutary effects including anti-inflammatory, antioxidant, antiapoptotic, and antithrombotic actions, and vasorelaxant, antidiabetic, and infarct-size–reducing properties. These pleiotropic actions may potentially contribute to the benefits conveyed by HDL. These mechanisms that involve the HDL proteome and lipidome have been extensively reviewed elsewhere.[15,31]

Anti-inflammatory Properties

Aside from RCT, the next best recognized HDL function is anti-inflammatory regulation. In contrast to its important positive effect on RCT, lipid-poor apoA-I does not possess several of the endothelial cell–protective and anti-inflammatory activities of HDL-C that are mediated by binding to SR-BI.[32] HDL reduces the expression of adhesion molecules and inflammatory markers in macrophages and endothelial cells.[33] HDL reduces tumor necrosis factor (TNF)-mediated induction of cell adhesion molecules (vascular [VCAM-1] and intercellular [ICAM-1]) both in cell culture[34] and in vivo models of atherosclerosis. HDL also inhibits the synthesis of monocyte chemo-attractant protein 1, responsible for recruitment of monocytes, dendritic cells, and T lymphocytes to sites of inflammation. Moreover, apoA-I treatment modulates macro-phage polarization from an M1 (proinflammatory) to an M2 (anti-inflammatory) pheno-type.[35] HDL also interacts with circulating leukocytes to limit inflammation through an ABCA1-dependent mechanism (for instance, apoA-I can inhibit adhesion through CD11b).[36]

HDL and the ATP-binding cassette transporters act at the level of hematopoietic stem cells (HSCs) to suppress HSC proliferation and the production of monocytes and neutrophils. HDL interacts with ABCA1/ABCG1 to promote cholesterol efflux in the bone marrow and to control levels and signaling of interleukin (IL)-3/granulocyte macrophage colony–stimulating factor. If HDL is lowered or ABCA1/ABCG1 is absent, there is excessive proliferation of HSC in hypercholesterolemia, resulting in monocy-tosis.[37] However, this HSC proliferation can be suppressed with liver X-receptor ago-nists. IL-23–mediated HSC mobilization from the bone marrow and extramedullary hematopoiesis in the spleen also result in monocytosis, but can also be prevented by increased HDL.[38]

Endothelial-Protective and Vasodilating Effects

HDL-C enhances production of nitric oxide (NO) from endothelial NO synthase (eNOS) through SR-BI activation[39] and can reverse the oxidized LDL-mediated decrease in NO production. SR-BI colocalizes with eNOS in the caveolae of endothelial cells, and interaction with HDL-C directly activates eNOS. ABCG1 is also needed in this pro-cess.[40] HDL-C is also capable of inducing eNOS synthesis, thus favoring vasorelaxa-tion.[19] Although apoA-I plays the major role, HDL-associated S1P may stimulate eNOS through activation of the lysophospholipid receptor S1P-I in endothelial cells.[19]

Ex vivo, HDL increases NO-mediated vasorelaxation in aortic ring preparations.[40] Moreover, HDL favors endothelial cell proliferation and migration by means of SR-BI,[41] which results in normalization of the dysfunctional atherosclerotic endothelium. Recombinant HDL (rHDL) enhances endothelial function in vivo in humans with normal cholesterol levels[42] and in individuals with low HDL-C levels.[43] Injection of HDL from healthy subjects into diabetic patients increased endothelial NO production, dimin-ished endothelial oxidant stress, enhanced endothelium-dependent vasodilation, and promoted endothelial progenitor cell–mediated repair.[44]

Antiapoptotic Actions

HDL attenuates TNF-α–induced[45] and oxidized LDL-induced[46] apoptosis of endothe-lial cells and macrophages by activating the Akt pathway and inhibiting proapoptotic Bax. HDL has been demonstrated to also inhibit apoptosis in macrophages through a pathway involving ABCA1 and ABCG1[47]; this action is crucial because apoptotic macrophages release metalloproteinases and cytokines, which cause plaque desta-bilization. S1P, which is mainly carried in the plasma by HDL, also possesses antia-poptotic properties.[48]

Antithrombotic Effects

Low levels of HDL-C have been associated with increased arterial and venous[49] thrombotic events. Intravenous infusion of apoA-I decreases acute thrombus forma-tion in an in vivo rat model of thrombogenesis.[50] The antithrombotic properties of HDL have been attributed to (1) increased NO production[39]; (2) enhanced prostacyclin synthesis (both apoA-I and lipids in HDL stimulate cyclooxygenase-2, the key enzyme in prostacyclin pathway) and simultaneous decrease in thromboxane A_2 synthesis; (3) moreover, large HDL particles can act as a surface on which the ability of activated protein C or S to cleave active factor V is enhanced[51] (thus inhibiting thrombin generation); (4) HDL has direct antiplatelet effects—in humans, infusion of reconstituted HDL decreases collagen-, adenosine diphosphate-, or thrombin-induced platelet aggregation[52]; (5) HDL shows some fibrinolytic properties because it upregulates tissue plasminogen activator.[53]

Antidiabetic Effects

HDL also potentially exerts antidiabetic effects. First, HDL directly improves β-cell insulin secretion through ABCA1 and ABCG1; in fact, deletion of ABCA1 in both mice[54] and humans (Tangier disease[55]) results in glucose intolerance. Moreover, cholesterol accumulation in β cells reduces insulin secretion, a phenomenon that can be rescued by β-cell cholesterol unloading, either by HDL-related RCT or the cholesterol-depleting agent methyl-β-cyclodextrin.[56] An acute infusion of reconstituted HDL increased plasma insulin levels and reduced plasma glucose levels in patients with type 2 diabetes (T2DM).[57] HDL also improves insulin sensitivity; interestingly, HDL activates adenosine monophosphate kinase via ABCA1 in endothelial cells, adipose tissue, and skeletal muscle,[56] and also increases glucose uptake in primary cultured myocytes from diabetic patients.[57] In fact, depletion of apoA-I in mice resulted in impaired glucose tolerance, whereas apoA-I overexpression increased insulin sensitivity.[58] Finally, reconstituted HDL infusion inhibited fasting-induced lipolysis and fatty acid oxidation both in vitro and in vivo in T2DM patients.[59]

Myocardial Ischemia-Reperfusion Injury

Another beneficial effect (although not directly related to atherosclerosis) is that HDL reduces myocardial ischemia-reperfusion (I/R) injury. HDL reduces the size of infarction in an I/R model; this effect is related to the presence of S1P.[60] Plasma HDL and reconstituted HDL have been shown to directly reduce infarct size ex vivo in isolated rat hearts[61,62] or in vivo in rabbit models.[63] In fact, elevated HDL-C reduces the risk and extent of PCI-related myocardial infarction and improves the long-term prognosis in patients.[64]

HIGH-DENSITY LIPOPROTEIN DYSFUNCTION

HDL loses its beneficial properties in certain pathologic situations (eg, acute situations such as acute-phase response[65] or influenza A infection,[66] or chronic conditions such as CVD[15] or diabetes[67]), which has been termed dysfunctional HDL.

In CVD, leukocyte myeloperoxidase (MPO) has also been associated with the generation of dysfunctional HDL, with proinflammatory properties.[68] Circulating HDL (with at least 2 apoA-I molecules in each particle) readily diffuses into the artery wall, specifically within MPO-enriched atherosclerotic lesions. MPO binds to one apoA-I α helix in that HDL particle, and promotes site-specific oxidative modification at residue Trp72 of the contralateral apoA-I helix.[69] In contrast to circulating HDL, most apoA-I in atheroma is not associated with the HDL particle; lipid-poor apoA-I in atheroma is cross-linked and oxidized at Trp72, thus resulting in a dysfunctional HDL particle, which is both proinflammatory and shows reduced ability to promote cholesterol efflux via ABCA1.[69] This oxTrp72–apoA-I can diffuse back to the plasma; in fact, the concentration of plasma oxTrp72–apoA-I is directly correlated with CVD, even after adjusting for HDL-C and conventional risk factors.[69] Furthermore, MPO-mediated oxidation fails to polarize macrophages from M1 into M2 phenotype[35] and also renders apoA-I unable to mediate beneficial changes in the composition of atherosclerotic plaques[35] (ie, MPO-oxidized apoA-I does not shift plaques into a less vulnerable and more stable phenotype).

Diabetes also causes HDL dysfunction, especially through nonenzymatic glycation of HDL-P. (1) Nonenzymatic glycation of apoA-I reduces ABCA1-dependent cholesterol efflux[70] and the HDL-mediated activation of LCAT.[70] (2) The usual HDL-induced inhibition of endothelial VCAM-1 expression is lost in HDL from diabetic patients, thus favoring the adhesion of macrophages to activated endothelial cells[44,71,72] and reducing the anti-inflammatory activity of HDL. (3) HDL from diabetic patients loses its vasorelaxant effects, owing to a reduced ability to stimulate endothelial NO production (thus decreasing endothelial-dependent vasodilation), and also mitigates endothelial progenitor cell–mediated endothelial repair.[73] (4) HDL from diabetic patients activates proapoptotic pathways while failing to activate antiapoptotic proteins in endothelial cells.[72]

There are other mechanisms explaining dysfunctional HDL in CVD. Chronic inflammation (atherosclerosis is also considered a chronic inflammatory status) elevates serum amyloid A (SAA) protein,[74] and SAA displaces apoA-I from the surface of HDL, thus generating free apoA-I, which is cleared faster by the kidney. Furthermore, oxidative stress is enhanced in CVD, which both reduces the levels of PON-1[75] and selectively oxidizes amino acid residues in apoA-I (such as Met, Cys, Tyr, and Lys), with the final result being a decrease in the antioxidant capacity of HDL particles.

Chronic kidney disease (CKD) is associated with low HDL-C and increased CVD. Two different studies have focused on the HDL proteome in renal disease. CKD patients undergoing dialysis have increased levels of the acute-phase inflammatory proteins SAA, lipoprotein-associated phospholipase A_2, apoC-III, antitrypsin, retinol-binding protein 4, and transthyretin in HDL, along with decreases in phospholipid and increases in TG content.[76,77] These changes correspond with impaired cholesterol efflux function[76] and impaired anti-inflammatory properties.[77] The decrease in PON-1 and glutathione peroxidase explains the lower antioxidant function; interestingly, the reduction in antioxidant activity of HDL is a predictor of CVD and overall mortality in CKD patients on dialysis.[78] These studies are suggestive of a link between HDL dysfunction and increased CVD risk in CKD.

The changes in lipid content also contribute to HDL dysfunction. The altered phospholipid composition of HDL results in an elevated sphingomyelin to phosphatidylcholine ratio, which increases HDL-P surface rigidity[79] (a key determinant of antioxidant activity of HDL)[80] and impairs HDL-P functionality. Moreover, diabetic dyslipoproteinemia is characterized by hypertriglyceridemia and low levels of HDL-C, with TG-enriched HDL resulting from a CETP-mediated interchange of TG from TG-rich lipoproteins to HDL-L/HDL-VL. A low CE/TG ratio indicates unstable HDL particles, which are rapidly cleared from the circulation, further decreasing HDL-P.

BEGINNING TO UNDERSTAND HIGH-DENSITY LIPOPROTEINS: WHY IS THE HIGH-DENSITY LIPOPROTEIN HYPOTHESIS SEEMINGLY FAILING?

As explained earlier, several modern studies have cast a shadow on the beneficial effect of HDL on CVD risk. Here a comprehensive hypothesis is formulated that may explain the atheroprotective effects of HDL assessed in both the "classical" and "modern" studies, which slightly curb enthusiasm for HDL. The authors propose that the focus on a surrogate measurement of HDL functionality, such as HDL-C, or the cholesterol content of HDL-P is not an accurate indicator of the beneficial properties of HDL. Thus, the focus should be more on quantitative measurement of

HDL (eg, HDL-P) and certain validated HDL functions (macrophage cholesterol efflux, antioxidant and anti-inflammatory properties), which truly reflect and are responsible for the actual beneficial effects of HDL. For instance, the relationship between HDL-C and CVD risk is partially confounded by the association between low HDL-C and high levels of LDL-P. In fact, data from the Framingham Offspring Study[81] demonstrate a significant disconnect between LDL-C and LDL-P in patients with low HDL-C levels; thus implying that a substantial portion of the excess CVD risk of patients with low HDL-C stems from an unrecognized excess of small, dense LDL-P containing less cholesterol than normal, which raises the issue of low HDL-C as a marker of athero-genic lipoproteins. It is recognized that HDL-C, apoA-I, and HDL-P are static mass-based measurements, and thus cannot represent a dynamic functional process such as RCT (or the anti-inflammatory, antiapoptotic, and antioxidant effects of HDL).

As previously stated, 4 recent lines of evidence have questioned HDL-C and apoA-I as relevant therapeutic targets. All of these drawbacks of the HDL hypothesis can be explained with the newly formulated hypothesis.

1. *Problem:* A recent study showed that some genetic variants in the endothelial lipase (EL) gene that raise HDL-C levels are not associated with a proportionally lower risk of myocardial infarction.[7]

   Possible explanation: The clinical relevance of HDL-P explains the results of this genetic analysis. Mutations resulting in reduced EL activity only increase HDL-C without actually increasing HDL-P; thus, patients with low EL activity may have higher levels of HDL-C but lower levels of HDL-P, which does not trans-late into reduced CVD risk.[7] On the contrary, the mutations resulting in reduced phospholipid transfer protein activity translate into reduced CVD risk because they result in an increased number of HDL-P.[82]

2. *Problem:* A subanalysis of the JUPITER trial has shown that HDL-C and apoA-I were associated with reduced CVD risk only among patients in the placebo arm. This beneficial association was lost among people on rosuvastatin 20 mg achieving very low levels of LDL-C.[8]

   Possible explanation: First of all, the JUPITER results are not supported by the Clinical Outcomes Utilizing Revascularization and Aggressive Drug Evaluation (COURAGE) trial; in fact, on-trial HDL-C levels in COURAGE at 6 months were associated with increased CVD risk after 4 years in the subgroup of 2193 patients who achieved LDL-C levels of 70 mg/dL or less[83] (although one must take into account that this analysis did not adjust for LDL-P or apoB). However, even only considering the JUPITER results one must take into account the clinical relevance of HDL-C versus HDL-P. Most importantly, as previously explained, HDL-P concentration has emerged as a predictor of CVD risk that may be superior to that of HDL-C in both population studies[84–86] and randomized clinical trials of lipid-modifying therapies.[87,88] In the Multi-Ethnic Study of Atherosclerosis (MESA), HDL-C was not associated with cIMT after adjusting for HDL-P and LDL-P; however, low HDL-P predicted higher risk of elevated cIMT regardless of HDL-C level,[85] even after adjusting for LDL-P. This finding is supported by a subanalysis of the Veterans Affair High-Density Lipoprotein Intervention Trial (VA-HIT)[87]; HDL-VS particles (with high capacity to accept cholesterol) were predictors of lower CVD risk (odds ratio [OR] 0.71, 95% confidence interval [CI] 0.60–0.84, $P<.01$), whereas the lower risk associated with HDL-M concentration was weaker (OR 0.82, 95% CI 0.70–0.96, $P<.02$), and for HDL-L/HDL-VL particles (with low capacity to regain cholesterol) it was nonsignificant. In fact, a recent analysis of the

JUPITER trial has shown that, even though HDL-C did not predict CVD risk in statin-treated patients, HDL-P did predict CVD risk in all patients (placebo and statin), even after adjusting for HDL-C levels.[88]

3. *Problem:* A recent meta-analysis and some population studies suggest that changes in HDL-C levels after initiation of lipid-modifying therapy are not independently associated with CVD risk.[9,10]

   Possible explanation: Only 5% of the total cholesterol carried by HDL-P is derived from macrophage cholesterol efflux,[25] so HDL-C may be an insensitive method for quantification of the antiatherosclerotic properties of HDL. Moreover, HDL-C does not represent many important HDL functions that are related to CVD risk, such as antioxidant, anti-inflammatory, antiapoptotic, and vasorelaxant properties. Therefore, HDL-C levels (or the change in them) may not be the proper parameter to assess adequately the contribution of HDL to CVD risk.

4. *Problem:* Recent clinical trials have shown that HDL-C–raising pharmacologic therapy increases HDL-C levels but does not reduce CVD events (eg, AIM-HIGH[11] and HPS2-THRIVE for niacin,[12] dal-OUTCOMES[13] for dalcetrapib, ACCORD[14] for fenofibrate).

   Possible explanation: Strategies that increase HDL-C without expanding the pool of HDL-P with its rich proteome/lipidome do not seem to be effective. First of all, the combination of statin and niacin does not increase the number of HDL-P[89,90] (niacin treatment in AIM-HIGH raised HDL-C by 29% but did not improve cholesterol efflux or the HDL anti-inflammatory properties[91]). Furthermore, dalcetrapib increases the CE cargo of each HDL-P but without effectively increasing the level of HDL-P. Fenofibrate (as used in the Action to Control Cardiovascular Risk in Diabetes [ACCORD] trial) has not been shown to increase the concentration of HDL-P; conversely, gemfibrozil (which reduced CVD risk in the VA-HIT trial[92]) is the rare example of a therapy raising the concentration of HDL-P (10%) and HDL-VS/HDL-S particles (21%). In addition, the methodological concerns about AIM-HIGH, HPS2-THRIVE, and ACCORD may have also played a role (see later discussion).

NONPHARMACOLOGIC STRATEGIES THAT POSITIVELY BENEFIT HIGH-DENSITY LIPOPROTEINS
Aerobic Exercise

Regular aerobic exercise moderately increases HDL-C by about 5%[93,94] (with increases in HDL-VL or HDL-L by 11%[95]). A minimum energy expenditure of 900 kcal per week (or 120 min/wk from physical activity was required to elicit changes in HDL-C.[94] Exercise duration per session was the most important element of an exercise prescription, more so than exercise intensity or duration. A meta-analysis of 25 studies estimated that for energy expended above this threshold, there existed a dose-response relationship; every 10-minute prolongation of exercise per session (ie, above 120 min/wk) was associated with a 1.4-mg/dL increase in HDL-C.[94] Exercise was more effective in raising HDL-C in subjects with initially total cholesterol levels greater than 220 mg/dL or if the body mass index was less than 28 kg/m^2.[94] In the first month of exercising the anti-inflammatory effects of HDL-C predominated; in fact after only 3 weeks of exercise, although HDL-C levels did not change, HDL-C preferentially converted to an anti-inflammatory state.[96] The exercise-induced improvements in HDL-C are mediated by exercise-induced increases in lipoprotein lipase (LPL) activity; interestingly, inactivity per se reduces LPL activity and, even just by reducing time spent in sedentary activities, the LPL activity is increased and HDL-C levels elevated.[97] Moreover, overweight patients who exercise and diet experience more HDL-C elevation than patients only on diet.[98]

Weight Loss

Weight loss has favorable effects on the lipoprotein profile. In obese patients, the loss of only 1 kg is associated with a 0.35 mg/dL increase in HDL-C concentration.[99] Weight loss of 5% to 10% of body weight results in approximately a 15% reduction in LDL-C, a 20% decrease in triglycerides, and an 8% to 10% increase in HDL-C.[100] Because LPL levels are reduced in acute caloric restriction but are greatly increased with established weight loss,[101] subjects actively losing weight experience an early and transient phase of HDL-C reduction and then HDL-C levels increase proportionally to weight loss when the weight is stabilized.[99,102] In 34 morbid obese patients, bariatric surgery was accompanied by a 20% decrease in weight, a 14% increase in HDL-C levels, a 42% raise in HDL-L particles, and an improvement in cholesterol efflux through ABCG1 and SR-BI.[103]

Alcohol Intake

Moderate alcohol intake (30–40 g daily, roughly 2 drinks in males and 1 in females) increases HDL-C levels by 5% to 15% and decreases CVD risk.[104–106] It seems to be ethanol per se that causes this modification in lipid profile, thus all alcoholic drinks can increase HDL-C.[106] In a recent meta-analysis of more than 16,000 patients, there was a J-shaped curve of alcohol consumption versus all-cause and CVD mortality[107] (maximal protection 18% and 22%, respectively); in another meta-analysis there was reduced CVD mortality in light (32% reduction) and moderate (38% reduction) drinking.[108] Notwithstanding, the benefits of alcohol consumption must be balanced against the risks (potential abuse, dependence, caloric intake, and heavy alcohol intake being associated with increased all-cause and CVD mortality[109]).

Tobacco Cessation

Among nonsmokers and light, moderate, and heavy smokers, a significant dose-response effect was present for HDL-C (reduction of 4.6%, 6.3%, and 8.9% for light, moderate, and heavy smokers compared with nonsmokers) and apoA-I (reduction of 0%, 3.7%, and 5.7% for light, moderate, and heavy smokers compared with non-smokers).[110] Tobacco cessation increases HDL-C concentrations (by 4 mg/dL in men and 6 mg/dL in women), apoA-I levels,[111] and HDL-P (especially HDL-L),[111] as early as 2 weeks after cessation.[112]

Diets

Mediterranean diet and diets rich in polyunsaturated free fatty acids (nuts, olive oil, and fatty fish such as salmon, trout, or sardines) increase HDL-C levels by approximately 3 mg/dL.[113] The PREDIMED study demonstrated that Mediterranean diet supplemented with olive oil or nuts increased HDL-C by 2.5 mg/dL in comparison with a traditional low-fat diet,[114] while also reducing LDL-C by 4 to 6 mg/dL and TG (only in the nut-supplemented arm) by 7 mg/dL. Furthermore, a Mediterranean diet caused a switch of the lipid profile to a less atherogenic pattern, with an increase in the number of HDL-P, especially of HDL-L,[115] and a decrease in LDL-P, specifically of the small, oxidized LDL-P in the nut-supplemented arm.[115] Most importantly, a Mediterranean diet reduced carotid atheroma burden[116] and CVD mortality.[117] Consumption of saturated fat reduces the anti-inflammatory potential of HDL and impairs arterial endothelial function. By contrast, the anti-inflammatory activity of HDL improves after consumption of polyunsaturated fat.[118] Even the specific consumption of fatty fish (fish containing high quantities of omega-3 polyunsaturated fatty acids, such as trout, salmon, tuna, or sardines) did not affect HDL-C, but increased HDL-P and shifted the distribution of HDL-P to a less atherogenic profile.[119]

Diets with low glycemic index both increase HDL-C levels[120,121] and improve HDL anti-inflammatory properties[96] while also reducing TG. In fact, considering glycemic index as a continuous variable, a reduction in HDL-C concentration of −0.06 mmol/ L per 15-unit increase in glycemic index in the diet was reported.[121] However, achieving nutrient adequacy via food-based dietary recommendations is difficult for an absolutely strict low–glycemic index diet because of limitations in foods allowed (eg, milk, fruits, and whole grains). Thus, long-term safety studies of this dietary pattern are needed before recommendations can be made.

PHARMACOLOGIC THERAPY TO RAISE HIGH-DENSITY LIPOPROTEIN CHOLESTEROL CONCENTRATIONS
Statins

In addition to LDL-C lowering, statins also do have a small effect on HDL-C levels. In a meta-analysis of 32,258 patients, it was shown that this increase was dose and statin dependent, with HDL-C increases ranging from 2.3% to 7.9%.[122] This effect did not correlate with the effect size of the LDL-C reduction. In fact, baseline HDL-C and TG levels were the best independent predictors of statin-induced HDL-C elevations.[122] Rosuvastatin exerts the most potent effect in increasing both HDL-C and HDL-P, an essential parameter regarding HDL functionality, as discussed earlier. In a double-blind study of 318 patients with metabolic syndrome, rosuvastatin increased HDL-P by 15% and HDL-C by 10% compared with placebo, and was more effective than atorvastatin in increasing both HDL-C and HDL-P.[123] Moreover, rosuvastatin increased both HDL-C and HDL-P in all patients, while atorvastatin was predominantly effective in patients with high baseline TG levels.[123]

This effect is partly due to a mild increase in apoA-I synthesis[124] and a reduction in CETP activity.[125] In addition, statin therapy seems to improve the effects of HDL on cholesterol efflux through SR-BI but not through ABCA1. Specifically, treatment with atorvastatin was accompanied by a dose-dependent increase in cholesterol efflux from hepatoma cells, an experimental model already validated for the SR-BI receptor.[126] Conversely, in J774 cells (an experimental model validated for ABCA1 receptor), incubation with statins reduced ABCA1-mediated cholesterol efflux to HDL,[127] which may be mediated by a statin-induced increase in miR-33 expression, thus reducing ABCA1 expression. However, whether such statin effects demonstrated under cell culture conditions are relevant in vivo remains unknown.

Fibrates

Fibrates, the agonists of the peroxisome proliferator–activated receptor α (PPAR-α), raise HDL-C levels by 10% to 20% while they reduce TG by 20% to 50% and LDL-C by 10% to 20%. It must be reiterated that gemfibrozil is the rare example of a drug that increases the level of HDL-C (by 7%) and, even more importantly, the concentration of HDL-P (by 21%).[87] Their mechanism of action is multiple.[128] Fibrates slightly increase the expression of apoA-I, ABCA1, and SR-BI, which directly causes an increase in HDL-C. Fibrates also decrease TG (by reducing VLDL synthesis and by activating LPL), leading to decreased CETP activity and thereby indirectly raising HDL-C. Therefore, TG reduction is an indirect way of increasing HDL-C, and the higher the baseline levels of TG, the more marked is the increase in HDL-C levels.

Several studies have been performed to assess the efficacy of fibrates on CVD end points, but the exact significance remains elusive. Positive results for gemfibrozil were reported from trials of participants with low HDL-C and high cholesterol and elevated TG levels. The primary-prevention Helsinki Heart Study showed a 34% reduction in CVD events with an 11% increase in HDL-C[129]; the benefits were more pronounced in the subgroup with TG greater than 200 mg/dL and HDL-C less than 42 mg/dL, in which there was a 72% reduction in CVD events.[130] However, as LDL-C was also decreased by 11%, these results could be attributed to LDL-C reduction. The secondary-prevention VA-HIT[92] clinical trial was the first trial to demonstrate that an increase in HDL-C concentrations reduced CVD events in patients. As LDL-C levels were identical in both study groups, the 22% reduction in CVD events could only be attributed to the gemfibrozil-mediated 7% increase in HDL-C levels. Of note, gemfibrozil treatment raised the concentration of total HDL-P (10%) and HDL-VS/HDL-S particles (21%); in fact the concentrations of these HDL-P achieved with gemfibrozil were significant, independent, inversely related predictors of new CVD events (OR 0.71, 95% CI 0.61–0.81, $P = .03$).

By contrast, the Bezafibrate Infarction Prevention (BIP)[131] and Fenofibrate Intervention and Event Lowering in Diabetes (FIELD)[132] clinical trials did not show a reduction in CVD events in the overall study population, but did reduce the primary composite end point in the prespecified subgroup with TG greater than 200 mg/dL and HDL-C less than 35 mg/dL.

Previously mentioned studies compared the effect of fibrate monotherapy with that of placebo. Only 2 studies (ACCORD and FIRST) investigated the effect of statin/fibrate therapy versus statin/placebo. For ethical reasons, all future novel lipid-lowering therapies for CVD event reduction will be started in conjunction with statins. The ACCORD lipid trial[14] studied in 5518 T2DM patients the combination of statin and fibrate versus statin/placebo; there were no significant differences in CVD events in the overall population but fibrates again decreased CVD events in the prespecified subgroup with TG greater than 204 mg/dL and HDL-C less than 40 mg/dL. The FIRST study[133] investigated fenofibrate/atorvastatin versus atorvastatin/placebo in patients with type IIb dyslipidemia and with controlled LDL-C. There was no difference in progression of cIMT between both groups; in post hoc analysis, the fenofibrate arm was favored in patients older than 60 years, with previous CVD, severe CVD (higher cIMT), and high TG. It must be emphasized that not all fibrates are created equal; unlike gemfibrozil,[87] fenofibrate has not been shown to increase the concentration of HDL-P, thereby not improving HDL metabolism. For a review of all the trials, see **Table 2** and other publications.[26] There is, therefore, solid evidence that fibrates significantly reduced CVD events when compared with placebo in subgroups of patients with reduced HDL-C and elevated TG, whereas there was no benefit observed in the subgroups without these characteristics or when combined with statin therapy.

Niacin

Niacin (vitamin B_3, at doses of 1–1.5 g) is the most effective therapy thus far for raising HDL-C. It increases HDL-C by 20% to 35%, reduces LDL-C by 15% to 20%, and reduces TG by 30% to 50%, while also decreasing lipoprotein(a). Of interest, niacin treatment does not increase the number of HDL-P but increases HDL-C exclusively, owing to an increase in the size of the HDL-P.[90] Niacin treatment also seemed to improve the cholesterol efflux and anti-inflammatory, antioxidant, vasorelaxant, and endothelial-protective effects of HDL-C in diabetic patients.[73,89]

Niacin initially showed consistent benefits in several small-scale clinical trials with and without statins using as outcome both clinical and imaging end points (atherosclerosis burden). For a review of all the trials, see **Table 2** and other publications.[26] However, great controversy has arisen over the last 2 years with the premature end of seemingly definitive trials combining statin and niacin therapy, namely the Atherothrombosis Intervention in Metabolic Syndrome with Low HDL/High Triglycerides: Impact on Global Health Outcomes[11] (AIM-HIGH) and the Heart Protection Study–2-Treatment of HDL to Reduce the Incidence of Vascular Events (HPS-2 THRIVE), both showing lack of effect of niacin treatment added to statins using CVD outcomes as primary end points. The AIM-HIGH study randomized 3300 statin-naïve patients who achieved LDL-C of less than 80 mg/dL on simvastatin + ezetimibe to a 3-year follow-up under additional 2 g of niacin or placebo, but failed to demonstrate a difference in CVD events between both arms. HPS-2 THRIVE enrolled 25,673 patients (32% with diabetes) with a follow-up of 4 years randomized to simvastatin + placebo or simvastatin/niacin/laropiprant (niacin causes flushing by binding to the PGD2 receptor and laropiprant inhibits this receptor, thus mitigating flushing), but also failed to demonstrate a difference in CVD events. Moreover, the niacin arm was associated with a 3.7% absolute increase in diabetes complications and a 1.8% absolute increase in new diagnoses of diabetes (25% increased risk of new-onset diabetes).

The design of both clinical trials may offer an initial possible explanation about the lack of effect of niacin. Several peculiarities of the AIM-HIGH study design limit its interpretation: (1) patients in the placebo arm received much higher doses of statins and ezetimibe (in a vain attempt to match the LDL-C levels between both arms); (2) small quantities of niacin (200 mg daily) were given to the placebo arm to maintain the double-blind status (regarding flushing), which explains why HDL-C increased 5 mg/dL in the placebo arm—thus, at the end of the study HDL-C levels were very similar (44 mg/dL in statin/niacin arm, 40 mg/dL in the statin/placebo arm); (3) the early termination of AIM-HIGH may have obscured a potential late benefit (eg, in VA-HIT the difference appeared after 3 years of follow-up); (4) it enrolled a very low-risk population (baseline LDL-C 71 mg/dL, TG 161 mg/dL, before randomization); (5) it is an underpowered trial (the REVEAL trial enrolled 30,000 patients and HPS-THRIVE enrolled 25,000, whereas AIM-HIGH enrolled only 3300 patients). Some additional comments should also be noted regarding HPS2-THRIVE. (1) The study only compared statin/placebo with statin/niacin/laropiprant, so it is certainly plausible that laropiprant is not really biologically inert, and plausible that some (or most) of the off-target effects observed in this trial may be related to laropiprant as opposed to niacin. In fact, mice knocked-out for PGD2 receptor exhibit accelerated atherosclerosis and thrombogenesis.[134] This issue could only have been addressed with a 2 × 2 factorial design. (2) The studied sample does not represent the actual population most susceptible to benefit from niacin treatment because it was at a very low risk (baseline LDL-C 62 mg/dL, HDL-C almost normal 44 mg/dL, TG 125 mg/dL, total cholesterol 128 mg/dL); it is highly unlikely that in real life clinicians would consider prescribing 2 g of niacin + laropiprant to patients with similar lipid profiles. (3) There was a large population heterogeneity because greater than 10,000 patients were recruited in China, and Asians are known both not to raise HDL-C by much in response to niacin and not to tolerate niacin or high-dose statins. Nevertheless, with 2 large outcome clinical trials being prematurely terminated for futility, niacin is unlikely to become a significant player in CVD risk-reduction strategies.

Additional hypotheses may explain the failure of niacin in this context. First and foremost, the combination of statin and niacin does not increase the number of HDL-P.[89,90] Therefore, strategies that increase HDL-C without expanding the pool

Table 2
Main randomized clinical trials involving HDL-C-raising drugs with their clinical and imaging end points

Study	Drugs	Patients Receiving Treatment, No./Total (%)	Elevation in HDL-C Levels (%)	Follow-up (y)	Outcomes
Nicotinic Acid					
Clinical outcomes studies					
CDP, 1975	Niacin	1119/8341 (13.4)	NR	6	Decreased (15%) nonfatal MI
CDP Follow-up, 1986	Niacin	1119/8341 (13.4)	NR	15	Decreased (11%) death
Stockholm, 1988	Niacin + clofibrate	279/555 (50.3)	NR	5	Decreased (26%) death; decreased (36%) CAD death
HATS, 2001	Niacin + simvastatin	38/160 (23.8)	26	3	Decreased (90%) first death, MI, stroke, or revascularization
AFREGS, 2005	Niacin + gemfibrozil + cholestyramine	71/143 (49.7)	36	2.5	Decreased (13%) composite clinical outcome of angina, MI, TIA, stroke, death, and CV procedures; decreased focal coronary stenosis (secondary outcome)
AIM-HIGH, 2011[11]	Niacin + simvastatin	1718/3414 (50.3)	25 (12)	3	No difference in primary end point (MI, coronary death, hospitalized, revascularization)
HPS2-THRIVE, 2013	Niacin + laropiprant	12,838/25,673 (50)	13	3.9	No difference in primary end point (coronary event, stroke, revascularization)
Imaging studies					
CLAS I, 1987	Niacin + colestipol	94/188 (50.0)	37	2	Decreased coronary atherosclerosis
CLAS II, 1990	Niacin + colestipol	75/138 (54.3)	37	4	Decreased coronary atherosclerosis
FATS, 1990	Niacin + colestipol	48/146 (32.9)	43	2.5	Decreased coronary atherosclerosis; decreased death, MI, or revascularization (secondary outcome)
CLAS Fem, 1991	Niacin + colestipol	80/162 (49.4)	38	2	Decreased femoral atherosclerosis

Study	Treatment	Ratio (%)			Outcome
CLAS IMT; 1993	Niacin + colestipol	39/78 (50.0)	38	4	Decreased carotid IMT (regression also observed at years 1 and 2)
SCRIP, 1994	Niacin + colestipol + gemfibrozil + lovastatin + aggressive lifestyle modification	145/300 (48.3)	12	4	Decreased coronary atherosclerosis; decreased frequency of new coronary lesion formation
ARBITER 2, 1994	Niacin + statin	87/167 (52.1)	21	1	No progression in atherosclerosis (carotid IMT)
ARBITER 3, 1996	Niacin + statin	87/167 (52.1)	23	2	Decreased carotid IMT
ARBITER 6, 2009	Niacin + statin vs ezetimibe + statin	187/336 (55.6), only 208 had follow-up study at 14 mo	18.4	14 mo	Decreased carotid IMT
Oxford Niacin Study, 2009	Niacin + statin	71	23	1	Decreased carotid wall area, as per MRI
NIA plaque, 2013[190]	Niacin + statin	145	6	1.5	No change on carotid wall volume, as per MRI
Fibrates					
Clinical outcomes studies					
Newcastle, 1971	Clofibrate	244/497 (49.1)	NR	5	Decreased (33%) MI
Edinburgh, 1971	Clofibrate	350/717 (48.8)	NR	6	Decreased (62%) death; decreased (53%) MI
CDP, 1975	Clofibrate: 1.6 g	1103/8341 (13.2)	NR	6	Nonsignificant decrease (9%) in nonfatal MI or CAD death (P>.05)
WHO Cooperative Trial, 1978	Clofibrate: 1.6 g	5331/15,745 (33.9)	NR	5.3	Increased (47%) death; Decreased (20%) incidence of CAD (mainly due to decreased [25%] nonfatal MI)
WHO Follow-up, 1984	Clofibrate: 1.6 g	5331/15,745 (33.9)	NR	13	Nonsignificant increase (11%) in death (P>.05)
HHS, 1987[129]	Gemfibrozil: 1200 mg	2051/4081 (50.3)	11	5	Decreased nonfatal MI or CAD death (34%, P<.02)

(continued on next page)

Table 2
(continued)

Study	Drugs	Patients Receiving Treatment, No./Total (%)	Elevation in HDL-C Levels (%)	Follow-up (y)	Outcomes
VA-HIT, 1999[92]	Gemfibrozil: 1200 mg	1264/2531 (49.9)	6	5.1	Decreased nonfatal MI or CAD death (22%, $P = .006$)
BIP, 2000[131]	Bezafibrate: 400 mg	1548/3090 (50.1)	18	6.2	Nonsignificant decrease in nonfatal MI or CAD death (9%, $P>.24$) Significant decrease if baseline TG >200 and HDL <35 (42%, $P = .02$)
LEADER; 2002	Bezafibrate: 400 mg	783/1568 (46.9)	11	5	Nonsignificant decrease (4%) in CAD and stroke ($P>.05$) Decreased (40%) nonfatal MI (secondary outcome)
FIELD, 2005[132]	Fenofibrate: 200 mg	4895/9795 (50.0)	1.2	5	Nonsignificant decrease (11%) in CAD death or nonfatal MI ($P = .16$) 24% decrease in nonfatal MI ($P = .01$) Nonsignificant increase in total mortality (19%, $P = .22$)
ACCORD[14]	Fenofibrate	2765/5518 (50.0)	1.8	4.7	No decrease in primary end point (major CV events) and secondary end points (major coronary events, stroke, CV mortality)
Imaging studies					
BECAIT, 1996[187]	Bezafibrate	42/92 (45.7)	9	5	Decreased progression of CAD
LOCAT, 1997[188]	Gemfibrozil	197/395 (49.9)	21	2.7	Decreased progression of CAD
DAIS, 2001[189]	Fenofibrate	207/418 (49.5)	8	3	Decreased progression of CAD in patients with DM

CETP Inhibitors

Clinical outcomes studies

Study	Intervention				Outcome
ILLUMINATE, 2007[141]	Torcetrapib + atorvastatin	7533/15,067 (50)	72	1	25% increase in CV events ($P = .001$); increased death (58%).
Dalcetrapib, DAL-Outcome[13]	Dalcetrapib + statin	7938/15,871 (50)	40	1	No difference in coronary event + coronary death + stroke

Imaging studies

Study	Intervention				Outcome
ILLUSTRATE, 2007[142]	Torcetrapib + atorvastatin	591/1188 (49.7)	61	2	No decrease in coronary atherosclerosis progression, as per IVUS
RADIANCE 1, 2007[97]	Torcetrapib + atorvastatin	450/904 (49.8)	54	2	No decrease in carotid atherosclerosis progression by IMT
RADIANCE 2, 2007[98]	Torcetrapib + atorvastatin	377/752 (50)	63	1.8	No change in maximum intima-media thickness
dal-PLAQUE[151]	Dalcetrapib + statin	64/130 (49.8)	31	2	No decrease in carotid wall (MRI) or macrophage infiltration (PET)

Therapies Specifically Increasing HDL-P

Study	Intervention				Outcome
ApoA-I Milano, 2003[5]	ETC-216 (Apo A-I Milano + PL)	45/57 (78.9)	NR	5 wk	Decreased coronary atheroma volume on IVUS
ERASE, 2007[6]	Reconstituted HDL (CSL-111)	111/183 (60.7)	NR	6 wk	No decrease in coronary atheroma volume on IVUS
Waksmann et al,[171] 2010	Autologous delipidated HDL	14/28 (50)	NR	2 wk	HDL-VS increased from 5% to 80% Atheroma volume was reduced by 12% ($P = .2$)
ASSURE, 2014[157]	Resverlogix	240/323 (75)	NR	26 wk	Reduction of 0.6% in atheroma volume as per IVUS ($P = .08$), which was significant if high CRP. Less vulnerability as per VH

Abbreviations: AHA, American Heart Association; CAD, coronary artery disease; CETP, cholesteryl ester transfer protein; CHD, coronary heart disease; CRP, C-reactive protein; CV, cardiovascular; DM, diabetes mellitus; HDL-P, high-density lipoprotein particles; HDL-VS, very small high-density lipoprotein; IMT, intima-media thickness; IVUS, intravascular ultrasonography; MI, myocardial infarction; MRI, magnetic resonance imaging; NR, not reported; PET, positron emission tomography; PL, phospholipids; TG, triglycerides; TIA, transient ischemic attack; VH, virtual histology; WHO, World Health Organization.
Adapted from Santos-Gallego CG, Rosenson RS. Role of HDL in those with diabetes. Curr Cardiol Rep 2014;16(8):512; with permission.

of HDL with its rich proteome/lipidome may not be an effective strategy. It is possible that shedding of atheroprotective proteins with niacin may result in a less functional HDL-P that does not improve cholesterol efflux or HDL anti-inflammatory properties,[91] thus providing a mechanistic hypothesis for these disappointing results. In addition, niacin treatment (without concomitant statin treatment) moderately enhances the capacity of serum HDL to promote cholesterol efflux from cholesterol-loaded THP-1 macrophages,[89] but statin therapy reduces cholesterol efflux through an miR-33–mediated decrease in ABCA1 expression.[127] Because all patients in both trials were actually treated with niacin on the background of statin therapy, the atheroprotective properties attributed to niacin may not be the same in statin-treated patients as those reported for niacin monotherapy.

Cholesteryl Ester Transfer Protein Inhibitors

Certain Japanese subjects with very high HDL-C levels attributable to low CETP activity were reported in 1989.[135] This discovery was the rationale for the development of several CETP inhibitors, including torcetrapib, dalcetrapib, anacetrapib, and evacetrapib. The first epidemiologic studies suggested that polymorphisms resulting in low CETP activity were associated with reduced progression of atherosclerosis,[136] but a longer follow-up of the same population contradicted this initial finding, showing more CVD events in those individuals[137]; since then, the evidence about the role of CETP is at best contradictory.[138,139] Torcetrapib was a promising agent because it increased HDL-C by 60%.[140] Unexpectedly, torcetrapib exhibited deleterious effects in humans. The Investigation of Lipid Level Management to Understand its Impact in Atherosclerotic Events (ILLUMINATE) clinical trial was a clinical outcomes trial studying the effect of torcetrapib on clinical events in 15,067 patients (45% with diabetes)[141]; it showed a significant increase in both CVD mortality and all-cause mortality despite an HDL-C increase of 72% and LDL-C decreases of 25%, while the 3 imaging studies confirmed atherosclerosis progression (using both intravascular ultrasonography [IVUS][142] and cIMT[143,144]).

The cause of this excess in mortality has been the subject of much debate, with 2 different hypotheses aiming to explain this unexpected finding. The first theory relies on the CETP inhibition strategy per se being deleterious because it increases HDL-C levels by increasing the cholesterol content within the HDL-P, not by increasing the concentration of HDL-P (thus not expanding HDL lipidome/proteome and not augmenting the HDL-VS, the main acceptors for macrophage cholesterol efflux). The second hypothesis is that CETP inhibition strategy is safe and useful (even some preliminary reports suggest that torcetrapib modestly improves the cholesterol efflux to HDL-L/HDL-VL[145,146]), but there was unexpected off-target toxicity of the specific molecule torcetrapib. In fact, torcetrapib resulted in activation of the renin-angiotensin-aldosterone system, increases in natremia, reductions in kalemia, and increases in blood pressure (in some patients up to 15 mm Hg)[141]; this vasopressor effect is driven by adrenal aldosterone and cortisol release in addition to endothelin-1 upregulation,[147] and in vitro studies showed that torcetrapib induced aldosterone and cortisol release from adrenocortical cells.[148] In support of this hypothesis, it is noteworthy that no effect on blood pressure or aldosterone levels was observed for dalcetrapib, anacetrapib, or evacetrapib, and that there is no association between CETP gene polymorphisms and blood pressure in 67,687 individuals.[149]

Dalcetrapib is the second CETP inhibitor tested in clinical trials. It increases HDL-C by 34%[150] but has demonstrated no improvement in CVD outcomes (although it was not harmful) in dal-OUTCOMES[13] in 15,781 patients, no reduction of atherosclerosis burden as evaluated by magnetic resonance imaging (MRI) or in plaque macrophage content as assessed by positron emission tomography in dal-PLAQUE,[151] and no improvement in endothelial function as per flow-mediated dilation in dal-VESSEL.[152] In the dal-ACUTE study, whereas HDL-C was increased by one-third, apoA-I and cholesterol efflux were increased by less than one-tenth,[153] further supporting the concept of dissociation between improvements in HDL function and HDL-C levels. This fact reinforces the previously explained notion that therapies that increase HDL-C without expanding the pool of HDL with its rich proteome/lipidome do not seem to be an effective strategy.

The Determining the Efficacy and Tolerability of CETP Inhibition with Anacetrapib (DEFINE) clinical trial[154] was performed to investigate the safety and efficacy of anacetrapib in 1623 patients with high CVD risk. After 76 weeks, anacetrapib increased HDL-C by 138% and reduced LDL-C by 40%, without any increase in CVD events or any sign of toxicity[154]; interestingly, anacetrapib treatment enhanced cholesterol efflux to HDL and the anti-inflammatory properties of HDL.[89] The Randomized EValuation of the Effects of Anacetrapib Through Lipid-modification (REVEAL HPS-3 TIMI 55) trial will be the outcomes clinical trial assessing the effectiveness of anacetrapib 100 mg in clinical practice in CVD patients in combination with statins; more than 30,000 patients have been enrolled, the follow-up is 4 years, and completion is expected by 2017. An interesting aspect of anacetrapib is the 40% reduction in LDL-C, so it is possible that anacetrapib improves CVD outcomes, but it will be difficult to demonstrate if this beneficial effect is due to the effect on HDL metabolism or to the additional lowering of LDL-C.

Evacetrapib is the most recent CETP inhibitor to be developed. Evacetrapib increased HDL-C by 129% (in monotherapy) or 88% (in combination with statins) and reduced LDL-C by 36% and 14%, respectively. The Assessment of Clinical Effects of Cholesteryl Ester Transfer Protein Inhibition With Evacetrapib in Patients at a High-Risk for Vascular Outcomes (ACCELERATE) phase III outcome trial is currently recruiting an estimated 11,000 patients at high CVD risk to be randomized to either evacetrapib 130 mg or placebo in addition to optimal lipid-lowering treatment.

Emerging Therapies Specifically Targeting the Concentration of High-Density Lipoprotein Particles

There is solid evidence that therapeutic strategies that increase HDL-C without expanding the pool of HDL-P are not effective in reducing CVD events. Therefore, there is an urgent need to develop new treatments that increase the concentration of HDL-P.

Resverlogix

Resverlogix (RVX-208) is a small molecule that acts as an apoA-I upregulator. The bromodomain and extra terminal (BET) protein inhibits apoA-I transcription; resverlogix inhibits BET, leading to enhanced apoA-I gene transcription and thus increased apoA-I synthesis. Resverloglix increased apoA-I mRNA expression, de novo apoA-I synthesis, and nascent HDL in vitro in hepatic cell culture; resverlogix also increased serum apoA-I by 60% and HDL-C levels by 97% in vivo in adult green monkeys, while simultaneously increasing cholesterol efflux via ABCA1, ABCG1, and SR-BI.[155] In an initial human study with 18 healthy volunteers, RVX-208 treatment increased apoA-I by 10%, HDL-C by 10%, cholesterol efflux by 11%, and HDL-VS by 42%.[155] However, these promising results were only moderately confirmed in the subsequent ASSERT study involving 299 statin-treated patients; RVX-208 showed a dose-dependent increase on apoA-I levels and HDL-C, with maximum increases of 5.6% and 8.3%, respectively.[156] HDL-P only increased by 5% (HDL-VS by 4%), which may not be enough to translate into improvements in CVD outcomes. In fact, the very recent ASSURE clinical trial did not show clear benefits. A total of 324 patients with CVD and HDL-C less than 39 mg/dL were randomized to RVX-208 for 26 weeks or placebo. There was no statistically significant difference in the primary end point (−0.6% change in percent atheroma volume as determined by IVUS, $P = .08$), but there was nonetheless significant reduction of atheroma in patients with high levels of C-reactive protein and also less vulnerability of the atheroma plaque as assessed by virtual histology.[157]

Apolipoprotein A-I Milano

ApoA-I Milano is a molecular variant of apoA-I characterized by the Arg(173)→Cys substitution caused by a rare point mutation (R173C), which allows for disulfide dimer formation and subsequent increase in the antioxidant properties of the thiol groups. The discovery that subjects from the Italian village of Limone sul Garda with very low plasma HDL-C levels (10–15 mg/dL) exhibited paradoxically low CVD risk led to the hypothesis that apoA-I Milano could be a more functional and beneficial variant of apoA-I.[158,159] In experimental animal models, apoA-I Milano has been shown to regress atherosclerosis in mice[160] and rabbits,[161] to change the atheroma plaque into a less vulnerable phenotype,[161] to reduce in-stent restenosis,[162] and to exhibit antithrombotic[50] and vasoprotective[163] properties. These beneficial effects have been initially confirmed in human patients. First, 47 patients immediately after acute coronary syndrome (ACS) received 5 weekly injections of apoA-I Milano, and IVUS revealed plaque regression of 4.5%.[5] Another study with injection of reconstituted HDL-C with apoA- I Milano was associated with reverse coronary remodeling and reduced atheroma burden.[164]

Direct infusion of recombinant high-density lipoprotein

Direct infusion of rHDL (a combination of apoA-I and phospholipids) has been shown to improve RCT[165] and to be endothelially protective.

1. In a human trial, Effect of rHDL on Atherosclerosis – Safety and Efficacy (ERASE),[6] 183 ACS patients received 4 once-weekly intravenous infusions of rHDL (CSL-111) containing apoA-I isolated from healthy humans combined with soybean phosphatidylcholine; atheroma burden by IVUS was the primary end point. There was an improvement in atheroma burden after rHDL compared with baseline; however, the treatment did not result in a significant change in atheroma volume compared with placebo, and there was a high percentage of liver abnormalities. Based on the results of CSL-111, a second-generation compound (CSL-112) is in development. In 44 patients with established CVD, CSL-112 increased the concentrations of HDL-P (especially HDL-VS), apoA-I, and HDL-C, while also elevating the cholesterol efflux capacity from macrophages.[166]
2. CER-001 is an engineered lipoprotein particle mimicking pre-β HDL (HDL-VS) and consisting of a combination of recombinant human apoA-I and 2 phospholipids. The CHI-SQUARE study failed to show a difference between placebo and CER-001 in the end point of nominal change in atheroma volume assessed with IVUS.[167] Two very recent proof-of-concept studies show that CER-001 had a statistically significant reduction in the carotid atheroma burden assessed by MRI in patients with homozygous familial hypercholesterolemia (MODE,[168] 23 patients) and hypoalphalipoproteinemia (SAMBA,[169] 7 patients).

Infusions of autologous delipidated high-density lipoproteins

Infusion of autologous delipidated HDL is another novel and promising strategy to positively affect HDL-P. Plasma from patients is collected and extracorporeally subjected to a process that selectively removes lipid from HDL; the resulting lipid-poor HDL, which resemble the apoA-I/phospholipid rHDL described in the previous section, are subsequently reinfused back into the patient. This strategy decreased diet-induced atherosclerosis in cynomolgus monkeys.[170] In an initial clinical trial with ACS patients, 7 once-weekly injections of autologous delipidated HDL reduced plaque volume by 12%, whereas placebo increased plaque volume by 3%. This difference was not statistically significant ($P = .2$) owing to the small sample size (only 28 patients). The concentration of HDL-VS increased in the delipidated arm by 28-fold (from an initial 5.6% to an impressive 79.8%), and this increase in the pool of HDL-P likely explains the impressive reduction in IVUS-determined atheroma burden.[171] Further larger studies that use this approach are currently being planned.

Apolipoprotein A-I mimetic peptides

ApoA-I mimetic peptides are 18-amino-acid peptides, which do not have sequence homology with apoA-I (containing 243 amino acids) but mimic the secondary helix-like structure of apoA-I without sharing primary amino acid homology. ApoA-I mimetic peptides are smaller than native recombinant apoA-I and are therefore easier to produce, a characteristic that is of particular interest for drug development. Several compounds have been developed by replacing a variable number of nonpolar amino acids with phenylalanine (F) or alanine (A) residues.

1. Intravenous L-4F inhibited lesion formation in diet-induced atherosclerosis in mice,[172] but did not increase HDL-C or change the anti-inflammatory properties of HDL in human patients.[173]
2. D-4F is the same peptide as L-4F, but is synthesized from all D-amino acids instead of L-amino acids, which confers resistance to intestinal peptidases, thereby allowing oral administration; in fact, oral D-4F protected mice from diet-induced atherosclerosis.[174] In humans, the administration of a single dose of D-4F to CVD patients did not elevate HDL-C but did improve the anti-inflammatory properties of HDL.[175]
3. To overcome the barrier of the cost of chemically synthesizing these peptides, a new variety of tomato genetically overexpressing the apoA-I mimetic 6F has been developed,[176] which also decreases atherosclerosis in a murine model.[176]
4. FX-5A is based on the initial compound 5A; intravenous administration of 5A complexed with phospholipids increased HDL-C, improved both cholesterol efflux and HDL anti-inflammatory capacity, and reduced atherosclerosis in an animal model.[177]
5. ETC-642 is an apoA-I mimetic peptide that has demonstrated reduced atherosclerosis in animal models, and has been shown to be comparable with human apoA-I with regard to cholesterol efflux and anti-inflammatory effects.[178]

SUMMARY

HDL were widely considered to be beneficial regarding CVD because there is an inverse correlation between HDL-C levels and CVD risk, because HDL exert atheroprotective effects in vitro and in animal models, and because initial proof-of-concept studies in humans show that infusion of HDL reduces atherosclerosis. However, recent data question HDL-C as a relevant therapeutic target because genetic and population studies have not universally shown the usual inverse correlation between HDL-C and CVD risk, and because clinical trials have not demonstrated a reduction in CVD risk with certain HDL-related pharmacologic therapies.

The main problem is that sensitive in vivo markers of HDL function are lacking. Given that the amount of cholesterol carried by an HDL particle is not likely to confer atheroprotection, serum HDL-C levels (or the change in them) may not be the proper parameter for assessment of the contribution of HDL to CVD risk. Besides, static measurements, such as HDL-C or apoA-I, do not accurately reflect a dynamic process such as RCT. Therefore, too much emphasis has been placed on HDL-C as a surrogate marker of HDL metabolism/action, when in fact HDL-C is a poor marker of HDL function. Thus, research should focus on more sensitive markers of HDL metabolism that truly reflect and are responsible for the actual beneficial effects of HDL, such as the concentration of HDL-P.

Finally, therapeutic strategies that increase HDL-C without expanding the pool of HDL-P, with its rich proteome/lipidome, do not seem to be an effective strategy to reduce CVD risk. Ongoing discussion of this topic should have some impact on the basic research about HDL metabolism and on the current and emerging therapies targeting HDL.

REFERENCES

1. Barter P, Gotto AM, LaRosa JC, et al. HDL cholesterol, very low levels of LDL cholesterol, and cardiovascular events. N Engl J Med 2007;357(13):1301–10.
2. Badimon JJ, Badimon L, Fuster V. Regression of atherosclerotic lesions by high density lipoprotein plasma fraction in the cholesterol-fed rabbit. J Clin Invest 1990;85(4):1234–41.
3. Badimon JJ, Badimon L, Galvez A, et al. High density lipoprotein plasma fractions inhibit aortic fatty streaks in cholesterol-fed rabbits. Lab Invest 1989;60(3):455–61.
4. Rubin EM, Krauss RM, Spangler EA, et al. Inhibition of early atherogenesis in transgenic mice by human apolipoprotein AI. Nature 1991;353(6341):265–7.
5. Nissen SE, Tsunoda T, Tuzcu EM, et al. Effect of recombinant ApoA-I Milano on coronary atherosclerosis in patients with acute coronary syndromes: a randomized controlled trial. JAMA 2003;290(17):2292–300.
6. Tardif JC, Gregoire J, L'Allier PL, et al. Effects of reconstituted high-density lipoprotein infusions on coronary atherosclerosis: a randomized controlled trial. JAMA 2007;297(15):1675–82.
7. Voight BF, Peloso GM, Orho-Melander M, et al. Plasma HDL cholesterol and risk of myocardial infarction: a mendelian randomisation study. Lancet 2012;380(9841):572–80.
8. Ridker PM, Genest J, Boekholdt SM, et al. HDL cholesterol and residual risk of first cardiovascular events after treatment with potent statin therapy: an analysis from the JUPITER trial. Lancet 2010;376(9738):333–9.
9. Ray K, Wainwright NW, Visser L, et al. Changes in HDL cholesterol and cardiovascular outcomes after lipid modification therapy. Heart 2012;98(10):780–5.
10. Briel M, Ferreira-Gonzalez I, You JJ, et al. Association between change in high density lipoprotein cholesterol and cardiovascular disease morbidity and mortality: systematic review and meta-regression analysis. BMJ 2009;338:b92.
11. Boden WE, Probstfield JL, Anderson T, et al. Niacin in patients with low HDL cholesterol levels receiving intensive statin therapy. N Engl J Med 2011;365(24):2255–67.
12. Landray MJ, Haynes R, Hopewell JC, et al. Effects of extended-release niacin with laropiprant in high-risk patients. N Engl J Med 2014;371(3):203–12.
13. Schwartz GG, Olsson AG, Abt M, et al. Effects of dalcetrapib in patients with a recent acute coronary syndrome. N Engl J Med 2012;367(22):2089–99.

14. Ginsberg HN, Elam MB, Lovato LC, et al. Effects of combination lipid therapy in type 2 diabetes mellitus. N Engl J Med 2010;362(17):1563–74.
15. Rosenson RS, Brewer HB Jr, Ansell B, et al. Translation of high-density lipoprotein function into clinical practice: current prospects and future challenges. Circulation 2013;128(11):1256–67.
16. Davidson WS, Silva RA, Chantepie S, et al. Proteomic analysis of defined HDL subpopulations reveals particle-specific protein clusters: relevance to antioxidative function. Arterioscler Thromb Vasc Biol 2009;29(6):870–6.
17. Toth PP, Barter PJ, Rosenson RS, et al. High-density lipoproteins: a consensus statement from the National Lipid Association. J Clin Lipidol 2013;7(5):484–525.
18. Nofer JR, Bot M, Brodde M, et al. FTY720, a synthetic sphingosine 1 phosphate analogue, inhibits development of atherosclerosis in low-density lipoprotein receptor-deficient mice. Circulation 2007;115(4):501–8.
19. Nofer JR, van der Giet M, Tolle M, et al. HDL induces NO-dependent vasorelaxation via the lysophospholipid receptor S1P3. J Clin Invest 2004;113(4):569–81.
20. Poti F, Simoni M, Nofer JR. Atheroprotective role of high-density lipoprotein (HDL)-associated sphingosine-1-phosphate (S1P). Cardiovasc Res 2014;103:395–404.
21. Vickers KC, Palmisano BT, Shoucri BM, et al. MicroRNAs are transported in plasma and delivered to recipient cells by high-density lipoproteins. Nat Cell Biol 2011;13(4):423–33.
22. Wagner J, Riwanto M, Besler C, et al. Characterization of levels and cellular transfer of circulating lipoprotein-bound microRNAs. Arterioscler Thromb Vasc Biol 2013;33(6):1392–400.
23. Rosenson RS, Brewer HB Jr, Chapman MJ, et al. HDL measures, particle heterogeneity, proposed nomenclature, and relation to atherosclerotic cardiovascular events. Clin Chem 2011;57(3):392–410.
24. Santos-Gallego CG, Ibanez B, Badimon JJ. HDL-cholesterol: is it really good? Differences between apoA-I and HDL. Biochem Pharmacol 2008;76(4):443–52.
25. Rosenson RS, Brewer HB Jr, Davidson WS, et al. Cholesterol efflux and atheroprotection: advancing the concept of reverse cholesterol transport. Circulation 2012;125(15):1905–19.
26. Santos-Gallego CG, Torres F, Badimon JJ. The beneficial effects of HDL-C on atherosclerosis: rationale and clinical results. Clinical Lipidol 2011;6(2):181–208.
27. Santos-Gallego CG, Giannarelli C, Badimon JJ. Experimental models for the investigation of high-density lipoprotein-mediated cholesterol efflux. Curr Atheroscler Rep 2011;13(3):266–76.
28. Khera AV, Cuchel M, de la Llera-Moya M, et al. Cholesterol efflux capacity, high-density lipoprotein function, and atherosclerosis. N Engl J Med 2011;364(2):127–35.
29. Li XM, Tang WH, Mosior MK, et al. Paradoxical association of enhanced cholesterol efflux with increased incident cardiovascular risks. Arterioscler Thromb Vasc Biol 2013;33(7):1696–705.
30. Doonan RJ, Hafiane A, Lai C, et al. Cholesterol efflux capacity, carotid atherosclerosis, and cerebrovascular symptomatology. Arterioscler Thromb Vasc Biol 2014;34(4):921–6.
31. Camont L, Lhomme M, Rached F, et al. Small, dense high-density lipoprotein-3 particles are enriched in negatively charged phospholipids: relevance to cellular cholesterol efflux, antioxidative, antithrombotic, anti-inflammatory, and antiapoptotic functionalities. Arterioscler Thromb Vasc Biol 2013;33(12):2715–23.

32. Feig JE, Hewing B, Smith JD, et al. High-density lipoprotein and atherosclerosis regression: evidence from preclinical and clinical studies. Circ Res 2014;114(1): 205–13.
33. Nicholls SJ, Dusting GJ, Cutri B, et al. Reconstituted high-density lipoproteins inhibit the acute pro-oxidant and proinflammatory vascular changes induced by a periarterial collar in normocholesterolemic rabbits. Circulation 2005;111(12): 1543–50.
34. Cockerill GW, Rye KA, Gamble JR, et al. High-density lipoproteins inhibit cytokine-induced expression of endothelial cell adhesion molecules. Arterioscler Thromb Vasc Biol 1995;15(11):1987–94.
35. Hewing B, Parathath S, Barrett T, et al. Effects of native and myeloperoxidase-modified apolipoprotein a-I on reverse cholesterol transport and atherosclerosis in mice. Arterioscler Thromb Vasc Biol 2014;34(4):779–89.
36. Murphy AJ, Woollard KJ, Hoang A, et al. High-density lipoprotein reduces the human monocyte inflammatory response. Arterioscler Thromb Vasc Biol 2008; 28(11):2071–7.
37. Murphy AJ, Akhtari M, Tolani S, et al. ApoE regulates hematopoietic stem cell proliferation, monocytosis, and monocyte accumulation in atherosclerotic lesions in mice. J Clin Invest 2011;121(10):4138–49.
38. Westerterp M, Gourion-Arsiquaud S, Murphy AJ, et al. Regulation of hematopoietic stem and progenitor cell mobilization by cholesterol efflux pathways. Cell Stem Cell 2012;11(2):195–206.
39. Yuhanna IS, Zhu Y, Cox BE, et al. High-density lipoprotein binding to scavenger receptor-BI activates endothelial nitric oxide synthase. Nat Med 2001;7(7): 853–7.
40. Tall AR. Cholesterol efflux pathways and other potential mechanisms involved in the athero-protective effect of high density lipoproteins. J Intern Med 2008; 263(3):256–73.
41. Seetharam D, Mineo C, Gormley AK, et al. High-density lipoprotein promotes endothelial cell migration and reendothelialization via scavenger receptor-B type I. Circ Res 2006;98(1):63–72.
42. Spieker LE, Sudano I, Hurlimann D, et al. High-density lipoprotein restores endothelial function in hypercholesterolemic men. Circulation 2002;105(12): 1399–402.
43. Bisoendial RJ, Hovingh GK, Levels JH, et al. Restoration of endothelial function by increasing high-density lipoprotein in subjects with isolated low high-density lipoprotein. Circulation 2003;107(23):2944–8.
44. Besler C, Heinrich K, Rohrer L, et al. Mechanisms underlying adverse effects of HDL on eNOS-activating pathways in patients with coronary artery disease. J Clin Invest 2011;121(7):2693–708.
45. Sugano M, Tsuchida K, Makino N. High-density lipoproteins protect endothelial cells from tumor necrosis factor-alpha-induced apoptosis. Biochem Biophys Res Commun 2000;272(3):872–6.
46. Suc I, Escargueil-Blanc I, Troly M, et al. HDL and ApoA prevent cell death of endothelial cells induced by oxidized LDL. Arterioscler Thromb Vasc Biol 1997;17(10): 2158–66.
47. Yvan-Charvet L, Pagler TA, Seimon TA, et al. ABCA1 and ABCG1 protect against oxidative stress-induced macrophage apoptosis during efferocytosis. Circ Res 2010;106(12):1861–9.
48. Kontush A, Therond P, Zerrad A, et al. Preferential sphingosine-1-phosphate enrichment and sphingomyelin depletion are key features of small dense HDL3

particles: relevance to antiapoptotic and antioxidative activities. Arterioscler Thromb Vasc Biol 2007;27(8):1843–9.

49. Deguchi H, Pecheniuk NM, Elias DJ, et al. High-density lipoprotein deficiency and dyslipoproteinemia associated with venous thrombosis in men. Circulation 2005;112(6):893–9.
50. Li D, Weng S, Yang B, et al. Inhibition of arterial thrombus formation by ApoA1 Milano. Arterioscler Thromb Vasc Biol 1999;19(2):378–83.
51. Griffin JH, Kojima K, Banka CL, et al. High-density lipoprotein enhancement of anticoagulant activities of plasma protein S and activated protein C. J Clin Invest 1999;103(2):219–27.
52. Calkin AC, Drew BG, Ono A, et al. Reconstituted high-density lipoprotein attenuates platelet function in individuals with type 2 diabetes mellitus by promoting cholesterol efflux. Circulation 2009;120(21):2095–104.
53. Mineo C, Deguchi H, Griffin JH, et al. Endothelial and antithrombotic actions of HDL. Circ Res 2006;98(11):1352–64.
54. Brunham LR, Kruit JK, Pape TD, et al. Beta-cell ABCA1 influences insulin secretion, glucose homeostasis and response to thiazolidinedione treatment. Nat Med 2007;13(3):340–7.
55. Vergeer M, Brunham LR, Koetsveld J, et al. Carriers of loss-of-function mutations in ABCA1 display pancreatic beta-cell dysfunction. Diabetes Care 2010;33(4):869–74.
56. Drew BG, Rye KA, Duffy SJ, et al. The emerging role of HDL in glucose metabolism. Nat Rev Endocrinol 2012;8(4):237–45.
57. Drew BG, Duffy SJ, Formosa MF, et al. High-density lipoprotein modulates glucose metabolism in patients with type 2 diabetes mellitus. Circulation 2009;119(15):2103–11.
58. Han R, Lai R, Ding Q, et al. Apolipoprotein A-I stimulates AMP-activated protein kinase and improves glucose metabolism. Diabetologia 2007;50(9):1960–8.
59. Drew BG, Carey AL, Natoli AK, et al. Reconstituted high-density lipoprotein infusion modulates fatty acid metabolism in patients with type 2 diabetes mellitus. J Lipid Res 2011;52(3):572–81.
60. Theilmeier G, Schmidt C, Herrmann J, et al. High-density lipoproteins and their constituent, sphingosine-1-phosphate, directly protect the heart against ischemia/reperfusion injury in vivo via the S1P3 lysophospholipid receptor. Circulation 2006;114(13):1403–9.
61. Calabresi L, Rossoni G, Gomaraschi M, et al. High-density lipoproteins protect isolated rat hearts from ischemia-reperfusion injury by reducing cardiac tumor necrosis factor-alpha content and enhancing prostaglandin release. Circ Res 2003;92(3):330–7.
62. Rossoni G, Gomaraschi M, Berti F, et al. Synthetic high-density lipoproteins exert cardioprotective effects in myocardial ischemia/reperfusion injury. J Pharmacol Exp Ther 2004;308(1):79–84.
63. Marchesi M, Booth EA, Rossoni G, et al. Apolipoprotein A-IMilano/POPC complex attenuates post-ischemic ventricular dysfunction in the isolated rabbit heart. Atherosclerosis 2008;197(2):572–8.
64. Sattler KJ, Herrmann J, Yun S, et al. High high-density lipoprotein-cholesterol reduces risk and extent of percutaneous coronary intervention-related myocardial infarction and improves long-term outcome in patients undergoing elective percutaneous coronary intervention. Eur Heart J 2009;30(15):1894–902.
65. Van Lenten BJ, Hama SY, de Beer FC, et al. Anti-inflammatory HDL becomes pro-inflammatory during the acute phase response. Loss of protective effect

of HDL against LDL oxidation in aortic wall cell cocultures. J Clin Invest 1995; 96(6):2758–67.

66. Van Lenten BJ, Wagner AC, Nayak DP, et al. High-density lipoprotein loses its anti-inflammatory properties during acute influenza A infection. Circulation 2001;103(18):2283–8.

67. Morgantini C, Natali A, Boldrini B, et al. Anti-inflammatory and antioxidant properties of HDLs are impaired in type 2 diabetes. Diabetes 2011;60(10):2617–23.

68. Zheng L, Nukuna B, Brennan ML, et al. Apolipoprotein A-I is a selective target for myeloperoxidase-catalyzed oxidation and functional impairment in subjects with cardiovascular disease. J Clin Invest 2004;114(4):529–41.

69. Huang Y, Didonato JA, Levison BS, et al. An abundant dysfunctional apolipoprotein A1 in human atheroma. Nat Med 2014;20:193–203.

70. Hoang A, Murphy AJ, Coughlan MT, et al. Advanced glycation of apolipoprotein A-I impairs its anti-atherogenic properties. Diabetologia 2007;50(8):1770–9.

71. Ansell BJ, Navab M, Hama S, et al. Inflammatory/antiinflammatory properties of high-density lipoprotein distinguish patients from control subjects better than high-density lipoprotein cholesterol levels and are favorably affected by simvastatin treatment. Circulation 2003;108(22):2751–6.

72. Riwanto M, Rohrer L, Roschitzki B, et al. Altered activation of endothelial anti- and proapoptotic pathways by high-density lipoprotein from patients with coronary artery disease: role of high-density lipoprotein-proteome remodeling. Circulation 2013;127(8):891–904.

73. Sorrentino SA, Besler C, Rohrer L, et al. Endothelial-vasoprotective effects of high-density lipoprotein are impaired in patients with type 2 diabetes mellitus but are improved after extended-release niacin therapy. Circulation 2010; 121(1):110–22.

74. Choudhury RP, Leyva F. C-Reactive protein, serum amyloid A protein, and coronary events. Circulation 1999;100(15):e65–6.

75. Nobecourt E, Jacqueminet S, Hansel B, et al. Defective antioxidative activity of small dense HDL3 particles in type 2 diabetes: relationship to elevated oxidative stress and hyperglycaemia. Diabetologia 2005;48(3):529–38.

76. Holzer M, Birner-Gruenberger R, Stojakovic T, et al. Uremia alters HDL composition and function. J Am Soc Nephrol 2011;22(9):1631–41.

77. Weichhart T, Kopecky C, Kubicek M, et al. Serum amyloid A in uremic HDL promotes inflammation. J Am Soc Nephrol 2012;23(5):934–47.

78. Kalantar-Zadeh K, Kopple JD, Kamranpour N, et al. HDL-inflammatory index correlates with poor outcome in hemodialysis patients. Kidney Int 2007;72(9): 1149–56.

79. de Souza JA, Vindis C, Hansel B, et al. Metabolic syndrome features small, apolipoprotein A-I-poor, triglyceride-rich HDL3 particles with defective anti-apoptotic activity. Atherosclerosis 2008;197(1):84–94.

80. Zerrad-Saadi A, Therond P, Chantepie S, et al. HDL3-mediated inactivation of LDL-associated phospholipid hydroperoxides is determined by the redox status of apolipoprotein A-I and HDL particle surface lipid rigidity: relevance to inflammation and atherogenesis. Arterioscler Thromb Vasc Biol 2009;29(12):2169–75.

81. Otvos JD, Jeyarajah EJ, Cromwell WC. Measurement issues related to lipoprotein heterogeneity. Am J Cardiol 2002;90(8A):22i–9i.

82. Vergeer M, Boekholdt SM, Sandhu MS, et al. Genetic variation at the phospholipid transfer protein locus affects its activity and high-density lipoprotein size and is a novel marker of cardiovascular disease susceptibility. Circulation 2010;122(5):470–7.

83. Acharjee S, Boden WE, Hartigan PM, et al. Low levels of high-density lipoprotein cholesterol and increased risk of cardiovascular events in stable ischemic heart disease patients: a post-hoc analysis from the COURAGE Trial (Clinical Outcomes Utilizing Revascularization and Aggressive Drug Evaluation). J Am Coll Cardiol 2013;62(20):1826–33.

84. Kuller LH, Grandits G, Cohen JD, et al. Lipoprotein particles, insulin, adiponectin, C-reactive protein and risk of coronary heart disease among men with metabolic syndrome. Atherosclerosis 2007;195(1):122–8.

85. Mackey RH, Greenland P, Goff DC Jr, et al. High-density lipoprotein cholesterol and particle concentrations, carotid atherosclerosis, and coronary events: MESA (multi-ethnic study of atherosclerosis). J Am Coll Cardiol 2012;60(6): 508–16.

86. Akinkuolie AO, Paynter NP, Padmanabhan L, et al. High-density lipoprotein particle subclass heterogeneity and incident coronary heart disease. Circ Cardiovasc Qual Outcomes 2014;7(1):55–63.

87. Otvos JD, Collins D, Freedman DS, et al. Low-density lipoprotein and high-density lipoprotein particle subclasses predict coronary events and are favorably changed by gemfibrozil therapy in the Veterans Affairs High-Density Lipoprotein Intervention Trial. Circulation 2006;113(12):1556–63.

88. Mora S, Glynn RJ, Ridker PM. High-density lipoprotein cholesterol, size, particle number, and residual vascular risk after potent statin therapy. Circulation 2013; 128(11):1189–97.

89. Yvan-Charvet L, Kling J, Pagler T, et al. Cholesterol efflux potential and antiinflammatory properties of high-density lipoprotein after treatment with niacin or anacetrapib. Arterioscler Thromb Vasc Biol 2010;30(7):1430–8.

90. Airan-Javia SL, Wolf RL, Wolfe ML, et al. Atheroprotective lipoprotein effects of a niacin-simvastatin combination compared to low- and high-dose simvastatin monotherapy. Am Heart J 2009;157(4):687.e1–8.

91. Khera AV, Patel PJ, Reilly MP, et al. The addition of niacin to statin therapy improves high-density lipoprotein cholesterol levels but not metrics of functionality. J Am Coll Cardiol 2013;62(20):1909–10.

92. Rubins HB, Robins SJ, Collins D, et al. Gemfibrozil for the secondary prevention of coronary heart disease in men with low levels of high-density lipoprotein cholesterol. Veterans Affairs High-Density Lipoprotein Cholesterol Intervention Trial Study Group. N Engl J Med 1999;341(6):410–8.

93. Kraus WE, Houmard JA, Duscha BD, et al. Effects of the amount and intensity of exercise on plasma lipoproteins. N Engl J Med 2002;347(19):1483–92.

94. Kodama S, Tanaka S, Saito K, et al. Effect of aerobic exercise training on serum levels of high-density lipoprotein cholesterol: a meta-analysis. Arch Intern Med 2007;167(10):999–1008.

95. Kelley GA, Kelley KS. Aerobic exercise and HDL2-C: a meta-analysis of randomized controlled trials. Atherosclerosis 2006;184(1):207–15.

96. Roberts CK, Ng C, Hama S, et al. Effect of a short-term diet and exercise intervention on inflammatory/anti-inflammatory properties of HDL in overweight/obese men with cardiovascular risk factors. J Appl Physiol (1985) 2006;101(6):1727–32.

97. Hamilton MT, Hamilton DG, Zderic TW. Role of low energy expenditure and sitting in obesity, metabolic syndrome, type 2 diabetes, and cardiovascular disease. Diabetes 2007;56(11):2655–67.

98. Wood PD, Stefanick ML, Williams PT, et al. The effects on plasma lipoproteins of a prudent weight-reducing diet, with or without exercise, in overweight men and women. N Engl J Med 1991;325(7):461–6.

99. Dattilo AM, Kris-Etherton PM. Effects of weight reduction on blood lipids and lipoproteins: a meta-analysis. Am J Clin Nutr 1992;56(2):320–8.

100. Van Gaal LF, Mertens IL, Ballaux D. What is the relationship between risk factor reduction and degree of weight loss. Eur Heart J Suppl 2005;7(Suppl L):L21–6.

101. Schwartz RS, Brunzell JD. Increase of adipose tissue lipoprotein lipase activity with weight loss. J Clin Invest 1981;67(5):1425–30.

102. Weisweiler P. Plasma lipoproteins and lipase and lecithin:cholesterol acyltransferase activities in obese subjects before and after weight reduction. J Clin Endocrinol Metab 1987;65(5):969–73.

103. Aron-Wisnewsky J, Julia Z, Poitou C, et al. Effect of bariatric surgery-induced weight loss on SR-BI-, ABCG1-, and ABCA1-mediated cellular cholesterol efflux in obese women. J Clin Endocrinol Metab 2011;96(4):1151–9.

104. Gaziano JM, Buring JE, Breslow JL, et al. Moderate alcohol intake, increased levels of high-density lipoprotein and its subfractions, and decreased risk of myocardial infarction. N Engl J Med 1993;329(25):1829–34.

105. Valmadrid CT, Klein R, Moss SE, et al. Alcohol intake and the risk of coronary heart disease mortality in persons with older-onset diabetes mellitus. JAMA 1999;282(3):239–46.

106. Mukamal KJ, Conigrave KM, Mittleman MA, et al. Roles of drinking pattern and type of alcohol consumed in coronary heart disease in men. N Engl J Med 2003; 348(2):109–18.

107. Costanzo S, Di Castelnuovo A, Donati MB, et al. Alcohol consumption and mortality in patients with cardiovascular disease: a meta-analysis. J Am Coll Cardiol 2010;55(13):1339–47.

108. Mukamal KJ, Chen CM, Rao SR, et al. Alcohol consumption and cardiovascular mortality among U.S. adults, 1987 to 2002. J Am Coll Cardiol 2010;55(13): 1328–35.

109. Klatsky AL, Friedman GD, Siegelaub AB. Alcohol and mortality. A ten-year Kaiser-Permanente experience. Ann Intern Med 1981;95(2):139–45.

110. Craig WY, Palomaki GE, Haddow JE. Cigarette smoking and serum lipid and lipoprotein concentrations: an analysis of published data. BMJ 1989;298(6676): 784–8.

111. Richard F, Marecaux N, Dallongeville J, et al. Effect of smoking cessation on lipoprotein A-I and lipoprotein A-I: A-II levels. Metabolism 1997;46(6):711–5.

112. Maeda K, Noguchi Y, Fukui T. The effects of cessation from cigarette smoking on the lipid and lipoprotein profiles: a meta-analysis. Prev Med 2003;37(4): 283–90.

113. Esposito K, Marfella R, Ciotola M, et al. Effect of a Mediterranean-style diet on endothelial dysfunction and markers of vascular inflammation in the metabolic syndrome: a randomized trial. JAMA 2004;292(12):1440–6.

114. Estruch R, Martinez-Gonzalez MA, Corella D, et al. Effects of a Mediterranean-style diet on cardiovascular risk factors: a randomized trial. Ann Intern Med 2006;145(1):1–11.

115. Damasceno NR, Sala-Vila A, Cofan M, et al. Mediterranean diet supplemented with nuts reduces waist circumference and shifts lipoprotein subfractions to a less atherogenic pattern in subjects at high cardiovascular risk. Atherosclerosis 2013;230(2):347–53.

116. Sala-Vila A, Romero-Mamani ES, Gilabert R, et al. Changes in ultrasound-assessed carotid intima-media thickness and plaque with a Mediterranean diet: a substudy of the PREDIMED trial. Arterioscler Thromb Vasc Biol 2014; 34(2):439–45.

117. Estruch R, Ros E, Salas-Salvado J, et al. Primary prevention of cardiovascular disease with a Mediterranean diet. N Engl J Med 2013;368(14):1279–90.
118. Nicholls SJ, Lundman P, Harmer JA, et al. Consumption of saturated fat impairs the anti-inflammatory properties of high-density lipoproteins and endothelial function. J Am Coll Cardiol 2006;48(4):715–20.
119. Lankinen M, Kolehmainen M, Jaaskelainen T, et al. Effects of whole grain, fish and bilberries on serum metabolic profile and lipid transfer protein activities: a randomized trial (Sysdimet). PLoS One 2014;9(2):e90352.
120. Frost G, Leeds AA, Dore CJ, et al. Glycaemic index as a determinant of serum HDL-cholesterol concentration. Lancet 1999;353(9158):1045–8.
121. Ford ES, Liu S. Glycemic index and serum high-density lipoprotein cholesterol concentration among us adults. Arch Intern Med 2001;161(4):572–6.
122. Barter PJ, Brandrup-Wognsen G, Palmer MK, et al. Effect of statins on HDL-C: a complex process unrelated to changes in LDL-C: analysis of the VOYAGER Database. J Lipid Res 2010;51(6):1546–53.
123. Rosenson RS, Otvos JD, Hsia J. Effects of rosuvastatin and atorvastatin on LDL and HDL particle concentrations in patients with metabolic syndrome: a randomized, double-blind, controlled study. Diabetes Care 2009;32(6):1087–91.
124. Schaefer JR, Schweer H, Ikewaki K, et al. Metabolic basis of high density lipoproteins and apolipoprotein A-I increase by HMG-CoA reductase inhibition in healthy subjects and a patient with coronary artery disease. Atherosclerosis 1999;144(1):177–84.
125. Chapman MJ, Le Goff W, Guerin M, et al. Cholesteryl ester transfer protein: at the heart of the action of lipid-modulating therapy with statins, fibrates, niacin, and cholesteryl ester transfer protein inhibitors. Eur Heart J 2010;31(2):149–64.
126. Guerin M, Egger P, Soudant C, et al. Dose-dependent action of atorvastatin in type IIB hyperlipidemia: preferential and progressive reduction of atherogenic apoB-containing lipoprotein subclasses (VLDL-2, IDL, small dense LDL) and stimulation of cellular cholesterol efflux. Atherosclerosis 2002;163(2):287–96.
127. Niesor EJ, Schwartz GG, Suchankova G, et al. Statin decrease in transporter ABC A1 expression via miR33 induction may counteract cholesterol efflux by high-density lipoproteins raised with the cholesteryl ester transfer protein modulator dalcetrapib. American College of Cardiology 2013 Scientific Sessions. San Francisco, California. March 9-11, 2013.
128. Staels B, Dallongeville J, Auwerx J, et al. Mechanism of action of fibrates on lipid and lipoprotein metabolism. Circulation 1998;98(19):2088–93.
129. Frick MH, Elo O, Haapa K, et al. Helsinki Heart Study: primary-prevention trial with gemfibrozil in middle-aged men with dyslipidemia. Safety of treatment, changes in risk factors, and incidence of coronary heart disease. N Engl J Med 1987;317(20):1237–45.
130. Manninen V, Tenkanen L, Koskinen P, et al. Joint effects of serum triglyceride and LDL cholesterol and HDL cholesterol concentrations on coronary heart disease risk in the Helsinki Heart Study. Implications for treatment. Circulation 1992;85(1):37–45.
131. Bezafibrate Infarction Prevention (BIP) Study. Secondary prevention by raising HDL cholesterol and reducing triglycerides in patients with coronary artery disease. Circulation 2000;102(1):21–7.
132. Scott R, O'Brien R, Fulcher G, et al. Effects of fenofibrate treatment on cardiovascular disease risk in 9,795 individuals with type 2 diabetes and various components of the metabolic syndrome: the Fenofibrate Intervention and Event Lowering in Diabetes (FIELD) study. Diabetes Care 2009;32(3):493–8.

133. Davidson MH, Rosenson RS, Maki KC, et al. Effects of fenofibric acid on carotid intima-media thickness in patients with mixed dyslipidemia on atorvastatin therapy: randomized, placebo-controlled study (FIRST). Arterioscler Thromb Vasc Biol 2014;34(6):1298–306.
134. Song WL, Stubbe J, Ricciotti E, et al. Niacin and biosynthesis of PGD(2)by platelet COX-1 in mice and humans. J Clin Invest 2012;122(4):1459–68.
135. Inazu A, Brown ML, Hesler CB, et al. Increased high-density lipoprotein levels caused by a common cholesteryl-ester transfer protein gene mutation. N Engl J Med 1990;323(18):1234–8.
136. Kuivenhoven JA, Jukema JW, Zwinderman AH, et al. The role of a common variant of the cholesteryl ester transfer protein gene in the progression of coronary atherosclerosis. The Regression Growth Evaluation Statin Study Group. N Engl J Med 1998;338(2):86–93.
137. Regieli JJ, Jukema JW, Grobbee DE, et al. CETP genotype predicts increased mortality in statin-treated men with proven cardiovascular disease: an adverse pharmacogenetic interaction. Eur Heart J 2008;29(22):2792–9.
138. Vasan RS, Pencina MJ, Robins SJ, et al. Association of circulating cholesteryl ester transfer protein activity with incidence of cardiovascular disease in the community. Circulation 2009;120(24):2414–20.
139. Ritsch A, Scharnagl H, Eller P, et al. Cholesteryl ester transfer protein and mortality in patients undergoing coronary angiography: the Ludwigshafen Risk and Cardiovascular Health study. Circulation 2010;121(3):366–74.
140. Brousseau ME, Schaefer EJ, Wolfe ML, et al. Effects of an inhibitor of cholesteryl ester transfer protein on HDL cholesterol. N Engl J Med 2004;350(15):1505–15.
141. Barter PJ, Caulfield M, Eriksson M, et al. Effects of torcetrapib in patients at high risk for coronary events. N Engl J Med 2007;357(21):2109–22.
142. Nissen SE, Tardif JC, Nicholls SJ, et al. Effect of torcetrapib on the progression of coronary atherosclerosis. N Engl J Med 2007;356(13):1304–16.
143. Bots ML, Visseren FL, Evans GW, et al. Torcetrapib and carotid intima-media thickness in mixed dyslipidaemia (RADIANCE 2 study): a randomised, double-blind trial. Lancet 2007;370(9582):153–60.
144. Kastelein JJ, van Leuven SI, Burgess L, et al. Effect of torcetrapib on carotid atherosclerosis in familial hypercholesterolemia. N Engl J Med 2007;356(16):1620–30.
145. Yvan-Charvet L, Matsuura F, Wang N, et al. Inhibition of cholesteryl ester transfer protein by torcetrapib modestly increases macrophage cholesterol efflux to HDL. Arterioscler Thromb Vasc Biol 2007;27(5):1132–8.
146. Bellanger N, Julia Z, Villard EF, et al. Functionality of postprandial larger HDL2 particles is enhanced following CETP inhibition therapy. Atherosclerosis 2012; 221(1):160–8.
147. Simic B, Hermann M, Shaw SG, et al. Torcetrapib impairs endothelial function in hypertension. Eur Heart J 2012;33(13):1615–24.
148. Hu X, Dietz JD, Xia C, et al. Torcetrapib induces aldosterone and cortisol production by an intracellular calcium-mediated mechanism independently of cholesteryl ester transfer protein inhibition. Endocrinology 2009;150(5):2211–9.
149. Sofat R, Hingorani AD, Smeeth L, et al. Separating the mechanism-based and off-target actions of cholesteryl ester transfer protein inhibitors with CETP gene polymorphisms. Circulation 2010;121(1):52–62.
150. de Grooth GJ, Kuivenhoven JA, Stalenhoef AF, et al. Efficacy and safety of a novel cholesteryl ester transfer protein inhibitor, JTT-705, in humans: a randomized phase II dose-response study. Circulation 2002;105(18):2159–65.

151. Fayad ZA, Mani V, Woodward M, et al. Safety and efficacy of dalcetrapib on atherosclerotic disease using novel non-invasive multimodality imaging (dal-PLAQUE): a randomised clinical trial. Lancet 2011;378(9802):1547–59.

152. Luscher TF, Taddei S, Kaski JC, et al. Vascular effects and safety of dalcetrapib in patients with or at risk of coronary heart disease: the dal-VESSEL randomized clinical trial. Eur Heart J 2012;33(7):857–65.

153. Ray KK, Ditmarsch M, Kallend D, et al. The effect of cholesteryl ester transfer protein inhibition on lipids, lipoproteins, and markers of HDL function after an acute coronary syndrome: the dal-ACUTE randomized trial. Eur Heart J 2014; 35(27):1792–800.

154. Cannon CP, Shah S, Dansky HM, et al. Safety of anacetrapib in patients with or at high risk for coronary heart disease. N Engl J Med 2010;363(25):2406–15.

155. Bailey D, Jahagirdar R, Gordon A, et al. RVX-208: a small molecule that increases apolipoprotein A-I and high-density lipoprotein cholesterol in vitro and in vivo. J Am Coll Cardiol 2010;55(23):2580–9.

156. Nicholls SJ, Gordon A, Johansson J, et al. Efficacy and safety of a novel oral inducer of apolipoprotein a-I synthesis in statin-treated patients with stable coronary artery disease a randomized controlled trial. J Am Coll Cardiol 2011; 57(9):1111–9.

157. Puri R, Kataoka Y, Wolski K, et al. Effects of an apolipoprotein A-1 inducer on progression of coronary atherosclerosis and cardiovascular events in patients with elevated inflammatory markers. American College of Cardiology 2014 Scientific Sessions. Washington, DC. March 29-31, 2014.

158. Franceschini G, Sirtori CR, Capurso A 2nd, et al. A-IMilano apoprotein. Decreased high density lipoprotein cholesterol levels with significant lipoprotein modifications and without clinical atherosclerosis in an Italian family. J Clin Invest 1980;66(5):892–900.

159. Sirtori CR, Calabresi L, Franceschini G, et al. Cardiovascular status of carriers of the apolipoprotein A-I(Milano) mutant: the Limone sul Garda study. Circulation 2001;103(15):1949–54.

160. Shah PK, Nilsson J, Kaul S, et al. Effects of recombinant apolipoprotein A-I(Milano) on aortic atherosclerosis in apolipoprotein E-deficient mice. Circulation 1998;97(8):780–5.

161. Ibanez B, Vilahur G, Cimmino G, et al. Rapid change in plaque size, composition, and molecular footprint after recombinant apolipoprotein A-I Milano (ETC-216) administration: magnetic resonance imaging study in an experimental model of atherosclerosis. J Am Coll Cardiol 2008;51(11):1104–9.

162. Kaul S, Rukshin V, Santos R, et al. Intramural delivery of recombinant apolipoprotein A-IMilano/phospholipid complex (ETC-216) inhibits in-stent stenosis in porcine coronary arteries. Circulation 2003;107(20):2551–4.

163. Kaul S, Coin B, Hedayiti A, et al. Rapid reversal of endothelial dysfunction in hypercholesterolemic apolipoprotein E-null mice by recombinant apolipoprotein A-I(Milano)-phospholipid complex. J Am Coll Cardiol 2004;44(6):1311–9.

164. Nicholls SJ, Tuzcu EM, Sipahi I, et al. Relationship between atheroma regression and change in lumen size after infusion of apolipoprotein A-I Milano. J Am Coll Cardiol 2006;47(5):992–7.

165. Eriksson M, Carlson LA, Miettinen TA, et al. Stimulation of fecal steroid excretion after infusion of recombinant proapolipoprotein A-I. Potential reverse cholesterol transport in humans. Circulation 1999;100(6):594–8.

166. Gille A, D'Andrea D, Easton R, et al. CSL112, a novel formulation of human apolipoprotein A-I, dramatically increases cholesterol efflux capacity in patients

with stable atherothrombotic disease: a multicenter, randomized, double-blind, placebo-controlled, ascending-dose study. Circulation 2013;128:A15780.

167. Tardif JC, Ballantyne CM, Barter P, et al. Effects of the high-density lipoprotein mimetic agent CER-001 on coronary atherosclerosis in patients with acute coronary syndromes: a randomized trial. Eur Heart J 2014. [Epub ahead of print].

168. Hovingh GK, Stroes ES, Gaudet D. Effects of CER-001 on carotid atherosclerosis by 3TMRI in homozygous familial hypercholesterolaemia (HOFH): the modifying orphan disease evaluation (MODE) study. European Atherosclerosis Society Scientific Meeting 2014. Madrid, Spain, June 2, 2014.

169. Kootte RS, Smits LP, van der Valk FM. Recombinant human apolipoprotein-A-I prebeta-HDL (CER-001) promotes reverse cholesterol transport and reduces carotid wall thickness in patients with genetically determined low HDL. European Atherosclerosis Society Scientific Meeting 2014. Madrid, Spain, June 2, 2014.

170. Sacks FM, Rudel LL, Conner A, et al. Selective delipidation of plasma HDL enhances reverse cholesterol transport in vivo. J Lipid Res 2009;50(5):894–907.

171. Waksman R, Torguson R, Kent KM, et al. A first-in-man, randomized, placebo-controlled study to evaluate the safety and feasibility of autologous delipidated high-density lipoprotein plasma infusions in patients with acute coronary syndrome. J Am Coll Cardiol 2010;55(24):2727–35.

172. Garber DW, Datta G, Chaddha M, et al. A new synthetic class A amphipathic peptide analogue protects mice from diet-induced atherosclerosis. J Lipid Res 2001;42(4):545–52.

173. Watson CE, Weissbach N, Kjems L, et al. Treatment of patients with cardiovascular disease with L-4F, an apo-A1 mimetic, did not improve select biomarkers of HDL function. J Lipid Res 2011;52(2):361–73.

174. Navab M, Anantharamaiah GM, Hama S, et al. Oral administration of an Apo A-I mimetic Peptide synthesized from D-amino acids dramatically reduces atherosclerosis in mice independent of plasma cholesterol. Circulation 2002;105(3):290–2.

175. Bloedon LT, Dunbar R, Duffy D, et al. Safety, pharmacokinetics, and pharmacodynamics of oral apoA-I mimetic peptide D-4F in high-risk cardiovascular patients. J Lipid Res 2008;49(6):1344–52.

176. Chattopadhyay A, Navab M, Hough G, et al. A novel approach to oral apoA-I mimetic therapy. J Lipid Res 2013;54(4):995–1010.

177. Tabet F, Remaley AT, Segaliny AI, et al. The 5A apolipoprotein A-I mimetic peptide displays antiinflammatory and antioxidant properties in vivo and in vitro. Arterioscler Thromb Vasc Biol 2010;30(2):246–52.

178. Iwata A, Miura S, Zhang B, et al. Antiatherogenic effects of newly developed apolipoprotein A-I mimetic peptide/phospholipid complexes against aortic plaque burden in Watanabe-heritable hyperlipidemic rabbits. Atherosclerosis 2011;218(2):300–7.

179. Miller NE, Thelle DS, Forde OH, et al. The Tromso Heart Study. High-density lipoprotein and coronary heart-disease: a prospective case-control study. Lancet 1977;1(8019):965–8.

180. Castelli WP, Garrison RJ, Wilson PW, et al. Incidence of coronary heart disease and lipoprotein cholesterol levels. The Framingham Study. JAMA 1986;256(20):2835–8.

181. Multiple risk factor intervention trial. Risk factor changes and mortality results. Multiple Risk Factor Intervention Trial Research Group. JAMA 1982;248(12):1465–77.

182. Lipid Research Clinics Program. JAMA 1984;252(18):2545–8.
183. Assmann G, Schulte H, von Eckardstein A, et al. High-density lipoprotein cholesterol as a predictor of coronary heart disease risk. The PROCAM experience and pathophysiological implications for reverse cholesterol transport. Atherosclerosis 1996;124(Suppl):S11–20.
184. Goldbourt U, Yaari S, Medalie JH. Isolated low HDL cholesterol as a risk factor for coronary heart disease mortality. A 21-year follow-up of 8000 men. Arterioscler Thromb Vasc Biol 1997;17(1):107–13.
185. Sharrett AR, Ballantyne CM, Coady SA, et al. Coronary heart disease prediction from lipoprotein cholesterol levels, triglycerides, lipoprotein(a), apolipoproteins A-I and B, and HDL density subfractions: The Atherosclerosis Risk in Communities (ARIC) Study. Circulation 2001;104(10):1108–13.
186. Luc G, Bard JM, Ferrieres J, et al. Value of HDL cholesterol, apolipoprotein A-I, lipoprotein A-I, and lipoprotein A-I/A-II in prediction of coronary heart disease: the PRIME Study. Prospective Epidemiological Study of Myocardial Infarction. Arterioscler Thromb Vasc Biol 2002;22(7):1155–61.
187. Ericsson CG, Hamsten A, Nilsson J, et al. Angiographic assessment of effects of bezafibrate on progression of coronary artery disease in young male postinfarction patients. Lancet 1996;347(9005):849–53.
188. Frick MH, Syvanne M, Nieminen MS, et al. Prevention of the angiographic progression of coronary and vein-graft atherosclerosis by gemfibrozil after coronary bypass surgery in men with low levels of HDL cholesterol. Lopid Coronary Angiography Trial (LOCAT) Study Group. Circulation 1997;96(7):2137–43.
189. Effect of fenofibrate on progression of coronary-artery disease in type 2 diabetes: the Diabetes Atherosclerosis Intervention Study, a randomised study. Lancet 2001;357(9260):905–10.
190. Sibley CT, Vavere AL, Gottlieb I. MRI-measured regression of carotid atherosclerosis induced by statins with and without niacin in a randomised controlled trial: the NIA plaque study. Heart 2013;99(22):1675–80.

Lipoprotein(a)
An Important Cardiovascular Risk Factor and a Clinical Conundrum

Marlys L. Koschinsky, PhD*, Michael B. Boffa, PhD

KEYWORDS

- Lipoprotein(a) • Apolipoprotein(a) • Atherosclerosis • Thrombosis
- Oxidized phospholipids • Coronary heart disease • Genetics • Risk factors

KEY POINTS

- Concentrations of lipoprotein(a) (Lp[a]) are genetically determined predominantly at the level of *LPA*, the gene encoding apolipoprotein(a) (apo[a]); significant differences exist between ethnic groups in the genetic architecture of *LPA* and the distribution of Lp(a) concentrations.
- Although the role of the low-density lipoprotein (LDL) receptor in mediating clearance of Lp(a) from the circulation has been a point of controversy, it is becoming apparent that Lp(a) concentrations can be affected by therapies that influence this receptor, namely, statins and inhibitors of PCSK9.
- The true mechanism or mechanisms by which Lp(a) promotes coronary heart disease (CHD) remain elusive, although increasing evidence points to a key role for oxidized phospholipids that are possible covalently linked to apo(a).
- Although screening of the general population for elevated Lp(a) is not recommended, several types of patients could benefit from these measurements, possibly to target Lp(a) for lowering but more practically at this time to indicate those patients who would benefit most from rigorous attention to modifiable risk factors.
- A major unmet need in the field is a clinical trial in which the cardiovascular benefit of lowering plasma Lp(a) is assessed prospectively; such a trial would only be feasible with the advent of therapies to specifically lower Lp(a).

INTRODUCTION

A great deal of attention has recently focused on lipoprotein(a) (Lp[a]), an emerging risk factor for coronary heart disease (CHD) and possibly for other cardiovascular diseases. For decades, this lipoprotein particle has been an enigma: its true biological

Department of Chemistry and Biochemistry, University of Windsor, 401 Sunset Avenue, Windsor, Ontario N9B 3P4, Canada
* Corresponding author. Office of the Dean, Faculty of Science, University of Windsor, Room 242 Essex Hall, 401 Sunset Avenue, Windsor, Ontario N9B 3P4, Canada.
E-mail address: mlk@uwindsor.ca

Endocrinol Metab Clin N Am 43 (2014) 949–962
http://dx.doi.org/10.1016/j.ecl.2014.08.002
0889-8529/14/$ – see front matter © 2014 Elsevier Inc. All rights reserved.

endo.theclinics.com

function unknown; its status as a cardiovascular risk factor tenuous; and its clinical utility entirely unclear. Important advances have occurred over the last several years in the fields of genetics, epidemiology, biochemistry, and pharmacology to give new impetus to consider and manage Lp(a) in the clinical setting. After a brief introduction to Lp(a) structure and heterogeneity, this review focuses on the most recent findings in these spheres.

LIPOPROTEIN(a) STRUCTURE AND HETEROGENEITY

Lp(a) consists of a lipoprotein particle that is very similar to low-density lipoprotein (LDL), which is covalently linked to the unique glycoprotein apolipoprotein(a) (apo[a]) by a single disulfide bond (**Fig. 1**).[1,2] Apo(a) is homologous to the fibrinolytic proenzyme plasminogen.[3] Apo(a) lacks the amino-terminal tail region and first 3 kringle domains of plasminogen, but contains multiple copies of sequences homologous to plasminogen kringle IV (KIV) as well as a single copy of a kringle V–like domain and an inactive protease domain. Of the 10 different types of KIV-like sequences in apo(a), 9 are present in single copy in all isoforms, while one of them (KIV$_2$) is present in multiple repeats of between 3 and more than 30 copies.[4,5] This copy number variation is encoded at the level of the individual alleles of *LPA* (the gene encoding apo[a]) and accounts for the isoform size heterogeneity seen in the human population.[6]

Another level of significant heterogeneity in Lp(a) is in plasma levels of the lipoprotein. Plasma concentrations of Lp(a) are relatively stable within an individual, varying little in response to prandial status.[7] However, plasma concentrations of Lp(a) vary remarkably between individuals, with a range of greater than 1000-fold between the lowest and highest expressers.[8] Lp(a) concentrations are primarily genetically determined[8]: indeed, there is a general inverse correlation between apo(a) allele size and plasma Lp(a) levels[9] owing to the reduced secretion rate from hepatocytes of larger apo(a) isoforms.[10] Although the contributors to and magnitudes of genetic control of Lp(a) concentrations remain topics of debate, it is clear that the *LPA* gene itself is the major contributor to variation in plasma Lp(a) concentrations, with the size of the gene itself having the largest contribution.[9]

Compared with other lipoprotein classes, Lp(a) concentrations are relatively resistant to changes owing to dietary, exercise, or drug interventions.[11] However, evidence for lowering of plasma Lp(a) concentrations by several existing and investigational drugs has emerged, as in later discussion.

GENETICS OF *LPA*

Much of the recent interest in Lp(a) has emerged from genetic studies. Two landmark studies from 2009 showed that genetically elevated Lp(a) concentrations (from either small *LPA* allele sizes[12] or the presence of single nucleotide polymorphism (SNP) variants strongly associated with plasma concentrations[13]) are a risk factor for CHD. Indeed, the results of these studies indicate that elevated Lp(a) is causally related to the development of CHD.[12] Another recent study further reported that elevated Lp(a) is the strongest genetically determined risk factor for CHD.[14]

Significant questions remain as to the quantitative contribution of specific genetic variants to Lp(a) concentrations. Earlier data indicated that *LPA* genotype determined the vast majority (>90%) of variability in Lp(a) concentrations, with most of this, in turn, being accounted for by *LPA* allele size.[15] More recent estimates of the contribution of allele size or SNPs have furnished a much lower number (30%)[16]; it is possible that these later findings are, in part, a consequence of a real-time polymerase chain reaction (PCR)-based genotyping method that measures the total number of KIV$_2$

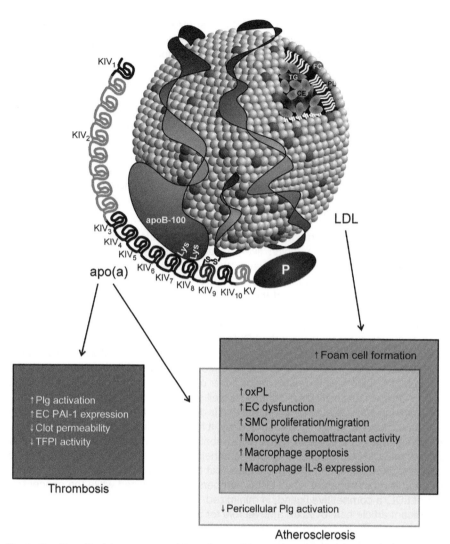

Fig. 1. Duality of Lp(a) structure and function. Lp(a) is composed of apo(a) covalently linked to the apoB-100 moiety of an LDL-like molecule. Apo(a) consists of multiple repeats of sequences related to plasminogen KIV and a single copy of kringle V (KV) and proteaselike (P) domains. The lipid content of the LDL-like moiety consists of a central core of triglycerides (TG) and cholesteryl esters (CE) surrounded by a shell of phospholipids (PL) and free cholesterol (FC). Lp(a) promotes both thrombosis and atherosclerosis: apo(a) promotes thrombosis because of its similarity to plasminogen (Plg), while LDL (and oxidized LDL) promotes atherosclerosis. Apo(a) also has several proatherosclerotic effects, shared with LDL/oxidized LDL, that are unrelated to it similarity to plasminogen. EC, endothelial cell; PAI-1, plasminogen activator inhibitor-1; SMC, smooth muscle cell; TFPI, tissue factor pathway inhibitor.

repeats in both alleles. Another complication of genetic studies is the differing genetic architecture of *LPA* in different ethnic groups, which likely underlies observed differences in the distribution of Lp(a) concentrations between different ethnic groups. In a multiethnic study, the same haplotype blocks were associated with Lp(a) concentrations in all 3 populations (South Asians, Chinese, and European Caucasians).[17]

However, the intronic variant (rs10455872) most strongly associated with allele size and Lp(a) concentrations in European Caucasians is not present in the other populations.[17] Another study in a Han Chinese population found that neither rs10455872 nor rs2798220 (encoding an Ile to Met substitution in the proteaselike domain and also strongly associated with elevated Lp[a] in Caucasians[18]) was associated with Lp(a) concentrations.[19]

It remains most likely that *LPA* allele size is the key driver of variation in plasma Lp(a) concentrations. Notably, there is no biochemical explanation for the association of any other polymorphism with Lp(a) concentrations, although this question has yet to be investigated directly. All *LPA* variants are in linkage disequilibrium with allele size, however.[17] Correlation of SNPs and haplotypes to allele size in a quantitative way will require allele-specific *LPA* genotyping for both SNPs and the length polymorphism.

LIPOPROTEIN(a) PRODUCTION AND METABOLISM

Variation in Lp(a) concentrations is primarily driven by differences in the rate of production, not catabolism,[20] which likely relates to the slower secretion of larger apo(a) isoforms.[10] It is notable, however, that very little is known about how Lp(a) is cleared from the circulation. Although the liver is the main organ responsible for Lp(a) catabolism,[21] the identity of the receptor or receptors that bind and internalize Lp(a) remains to be definitively established. In vitro studies point to a role for both the LDL receptor (LDLR) and the plasminogen receptors.[22] Studies conducted in mice or human subjects lacking the LDLR suggest against a major role for the LDLR in Lp(a) clearance, while still revealing a contribution of this receptor.[21,23] The effect of statins on Lp(a) concentrations has been controversial, again in keeping with the notion that LDLR levels are not a major driver of Lp(a) clearance. On the other hand, some studies in relatively large cohorts as well as a meta-analysis showed a measurable lowering effect of statins, albeit one that is dwarfed by the effect of these drugs on LDL-cholesterol (LDL-C).[24–26] Most recently, it has been demonstrated that inhibitory antibodies against proprotein convertase subtilisin/kexin type (PCSK9), a factor that diminishes LDLR numbers on the surface of hepatocytes, markedly decrease plasma Lp(a) concentrations.[27,28] Thus, it appears that the LDLR plays a role in Lp(a) catabolism that is most apparent when LDLR numbers are maximized while the concentration of LDL, a competitive ligand, is minimized.

A recent article has revealed a novel role for scavenger receptor-B1 (SR-B1) as an Lp(a) receptor.[29] SR-B1 mediates uptake of protein and, predominantly, neutral lipid from Lp(a). Knockout or overexpression of SR-B1 in mice clearly affects clearance of Lp(a), but the quantitative details clearly show that receptors other than SR-B1 play a role. The relative contribution of SR-B1 to Lp(a) catabolism remains to be clearly defined, and it will be interesting to determine if cholesteryl ester–depleted Lp(a) is targeted for preferential clearance and has any biological effects.

PATHOGENIC MECHANISMS OF LIPOPROTEIN(a)

The duality of Lp(a) structure that is readily apparent has given rise to the concept of a duality in the pathogenic effects of Lp(a), where the LDL-like moiety of Lp(a) serves to promote atherosclerosis, whereas the plasminogen-like apo(a) molecule promotes thrombosis by interfering with fibrinolysis (see **Fig. 1**). Although both of these effects have been documented for Lp(a),[30,31] extensive investigations have revealed many more facets than this simple model can account for. More specifically, several additional functions of apo(a) that do not necessarily arise from its similarity to plasminogen have emerged (see **Fig. 1**). These functions include initiation of signaling pathways in macrophages[32] and vascular endothelial cells,[33,34] resulting in proathero-genic changes in cell phenotype and gene expression.

Although a unifying mechanism underlying these unique proatherogenic effects of Lp(a) has yet to be conclusively demonstrated, a tantalizing possibility is that these effects may be attributable to modification of the particle by oxidized phospholipids (oxPL). In the EPIC-Norfolk study, oxidation modification of Lp(a) has been linked to CHD events and contributes additional predictive value to the suite of traditional CHD risk factors.[35] Moreover, the relationship of OxPL/apoB and Lp(a) to fatal and nonfatal CHD was accentuated in the highest tertiles of each, suggesting that they can provide independent information for risk prediction.[35]

Clinical studies have shown that Lp(a) is a preferential carrier of oxPL compared with LDL.[36] At least some of this is due to the ability of oxPL to become covalently linked to apo(a).[37] The oxPL, in turn, may act as ligands for cell-surface receptors, such as CD36, and Toll-like receptor 2 to initiate intracellular signaling cascades.[32] Interestingly, it has been reported recently that the addition of oxPL to apo(a) depends on an intact lysine-binding site in KIV_{10}.[38] Work in transgenic mice from almost 20 years ago showed that the lack of this site prevented the fatty-streak formation observed in mice overexpressing wild-type human apo(a).[39] More extensive structure-function studies will need to be undertaken to explore the importance of this lysine binding site and oxPL addition on the range of harmful effects of apo(a)/Lp(a).

Most recently, it has been reported that monocyte chemoattractant protein-1 (MCP-1), which is a proatherosclerotic molecule required for monocyte recruitment and migration across the vascular endothelium,[40] is carried by Lp(a) in human plasma.[41] In vitro, the binding interaction can be inhibited by E06, a monoclonal antibody against oxPL; this suggests that the oxPL modification of Lp(a) is essential for the binding of MCP-1. Overall, it is reasonable to speculate that the oxPL modification of Lp(a) contributes to its atherogenicity through the proinflammatory effects that are associated with oxPL; the association with Lp(a) allows these molecules to be targeted to the site of developing lesions.

ELEVATED PLASMA LIPOPROTEIN(a) CONCENTRATIONS AS A RISK FACTOR FOR VASCULAR DISEASE

It is well-established from retrospective case-control studies, prospective studies, and Mendelian randomization studies that elevated plasma Lp(a) is a risk factor for the development of CHD.[9] Most of the studies have focused on the influence of Lp(a) on a first occurrence of a coronary event. Some recent studies have sought to define whether elevated Lp(a) predicts the occurrence of events in patients with established disease. In a secondary prevention study that encompassed 18,979 subjects, Lp(a) in the highest quintile was associated with risk for subsequent events, although this relationship was lost for subjects with low LDL-C.[42] In the LIPID study, in which patients with a previous coronary event were randomized to statin or placebo, elevated Lp(a) (in the top quintile) was associated with risk for a variety of different cardiovascular endpoints.[43] In addition, in some patients, Lp(a) had increased after 1 year, and this was also associated with events.[43]

An important question is whether elevated Lp(a) remains a risk factor even in the face of aggressive lowering of LDL-C by statins. Analysis of data from the Justification for the Use of Statins in Prevention (JUPITER) trial did show a significant residual risk attributable to elevated Lp(a) in rosuvastatin-treated patients.[44] Thus, it appears reasonable at this time to consider the contribution of Lp(a) to a patient's risk even if the patient has existing disease and/or is receiving optimal lipid-lowering therapy.

Another longstanding question concerns whether small apo(a) isoforms are a risk factor independent of their association with elevated plasma concentrations of Lp(a). There are some biochemical data to suggest that small isoforms are more anti-fibrinolytic.[31] In the PROCARDIS study, adjustment for apo(a) isoform size did not alter the association of Lp(a) concentrations with CHD[13]; moreover, although small apo(a) isoforms were associated with increased risk, this association was abolished after adjustment for Lp(a) concentrations.

Two recent genetic studies have revealed that genetically elevated Lp(a) concentrations are associated with increased occurrence of aortic valve stenosis.[45,46] This disorder involves valvular calcification and is etiologically distinct from atherosclerosis, although it shares some common risk factors. Importantly, both studies demonstrated that elevated Lp(a) concentrations are in fact causal for aortic valve stenosis, as opposed to merely being a marker. The role of Lp(a) in the disease process is unknown, although Lp(a) appears to be deposited at sites of developing calcific valvular disease.

The ability of apo(a)/Lp(a) to inhibit fibrinolysis strongly suggests that elevated Lp(a) may pose a risk for pure thrombotic disorders such as venous thromboembolism. Although there have been discrepant results reported in the past, 3 recent, large, studies each also assessing *LPA* genotype at SNPs strongly associated with Lp(a) levels have concluded that no relationship between elevated Lp(a) and venous thromboembolism exists.[47–49] One study argued that this is evidence against a role for Lp(a) in the thrombotic complications of atherosclerosis.[47] There are, however, notable differences between the thrombi in arterial and venous compartments, with arterial thrombi being more platelet-rich, fibrin-poor, and initiated by the thrombogenic contents of the atherosclerotic core. Notably, a series of studies by Undas and co-workers[50] have shown that elevated Lp(a) is associated with reduced clot permeability and altered fibrin structure of plasma clots ex vivo.[51] In addition, Kardys and coworkers[52] found, in patients that had undergone percutaneous interventions, that elevated Lp(a) was associated with the incidence of major adverse coronary events within 1 year of the procedure, but not thereafter. One interpretation of these findings might be that they reflect the antifibrinolytic properties of Lp(a) because the early complications would be largely thrombotic in nature.

As surrogate markers of atherosclerosis become more specific and informative, the opportunity exists to more directly evaluate the role of Lp(a) in the atherosclerotic process itself. One such marker is coronary artery calcification (CAC), which is measured by computed tomography and is a sensitive indicator of preclinical atherosclerosis. The available data on the relationship between Lp(a) concentrations and CAC are conflicting. Studies have shown a positive correlation in large cohorts of European Caucasians or Asians,[53,54] although a smaller study found the Lp(a) was predictive of CAC only in Southeast Asians but not in European Caucasians.[55] Another study in a large cohort of European Caucasians found that although elevated Lp(a) correlated with increased CAC scores, Lp(a) was inferior to LDL-C or related measures,[56] the opposite of another study in a similar cohort.[53] Another study found that Lp(a) was only predictive of CAC in women with type 2 diabetes mellitus, but was not in women without diabetes or in men.[57] Clearly, additional studies are required to uncover the reasons for these discrepant findings and to determine the true relationship between elevated Lp(a) and subclinical atherosclerosis.

UTILITY OF LIPOPROTEIN(a) IN CLINICAL PRACTICE

Questions commonly posed by clinicians regarding the use of Lp(a) in clinical settings include the following: In which patients should Lp(a) levels be determined? How should Lp(a) concentrations be measured? What treatment strategy should be used for patients with elevated Lp(a) levels?

There is general agreement that measurement of Lp(a) in the general population is unnecessary.[58] However, there are specific clinical circumstances under which Lp(a) levels should be determined. These clinical circumstances are summarized in **Box 1**. Based on the current level of understanding, there is no additional benefit to the measurement of Lp(a) isoform size; this reflects the lack of evidence to suggest a role for apo(a) isoform size in CHD that is independent of the inverse relationship with Lp(a) levels.[59]

Because Lp(a) levels are genetically determined, it is suggested that a single measurement should be sufficient unless strategies are used that lower Lp(a) levels; in the latter case, response to treatment can be monitored through repeated measurement. An Lp(a) level above the 75th percentile has been taken as a decision point[58]; in Caucasian populations this corresponds to approximately 30 mg/dL. It is important to note that 30 mg/dL has been used in numerous epidemiologic studies to define elevated Lp(a) levels and is the most commonly used value used in clinical practice.[60] However, it must be recognized that this decision point might be expected to vary in different ethnic groups: in the Black population, for example, 30 mg/dL corresponds roughly to the 50th percentile,[58] although this cut-point still predicts risk for CHD in this population.[61] The Copenhagen Heart Study data reported greatly increased risk conferred by extreme Lp(a) concentrations greater than the 80th percentile of the study population (>approximately 50 mg/dL).[62] It has been suggested Lp(a) levels in excess of this value should be used to reclassify individuals into a higher risk category. This reclassification would include more aggressive LDL-lowering in this group, as well as the inclusion of niacin treatment as recommended by the European Atherosclerosis Society guidelines[63]; note that these recommendations are not universally accepted.[64]

As such, there is arguably no clearly defined cutoff point for the assessment of Lp(a) in CHD risk. The lack of this cutoff coupled with the lack of common reference materials for Lp(a) measurement and reporting of Lp(a) concentrations in different units, makes interlaboratory comparisons difficult. Although it is preferable to report Lp(a) measurements in molar concentrations (nmol/L) versus mass concentrations (mg/dL), many commercially available assays provide values in mass concentrations. A conversion factor of 3.17 (ie, 1 mg/mL of Lp[a] corresponds approximately to 3.17 nmol/L) has been suggested by the Lp(a) standardization group,[65] although a value of 2.4 has also been suggested[58]; using this latter value, 30 mg/dL converts to 72 nmol/L, which is a close approximation of the 75th percentile in Caucasian populations.[66] The ideal conversion factor will, of course, vary depending on the apo(a) isoform size present in the subject, so the suggested conversion factors are

---

Box 1
Patients in whom measurement of plasma lipoprotein(a) concentrations should be considered

- Patients with premature CHD in the absence of other risk factors
- Patients with a strong family history of premature CHD
- Patients who exhibit resistance to LDL lowering by statins
- Patients with recurrent restenosis or rapid disease progression with other risk factors controlled
- Patients with intermediate risk profiles[a]

[a] For example, 10-year Framingham risk score of 5%–19% or a CHD risk equivalent,[70] Lp(a) levels greater than 50 mg/dL would warrant reclassification into a higher risk category.[70]

necessarily average values. Another assay, the Vertical Auto Profile reports an Lp(a)-cholesterol value whereby 10 mg/dL (approximately the 75th percentile[67]) is the upper limit of normal.[68] Discrepant results have been reported for the relationship between Lp(a)-cholesterol and risk for cardiovascular disease,[67,69] and it has been suggested that measures of Lp(a)-cholesterol and Lp(a) particle concentration may be complementary.[68]

Based on the foregoing discussion, the authors' recommendations for Lp(a) concentrations above which intervention should be considered are as follows: 30 mg/dL (mass concentration); 75 nmol/L (particle concentration); and 10 mg/dL (Lp[a]-cholesterol).

Although there is no pharmacotherapy approved for use that specifically lowers Lp(a), in the subset of patients identified in **Box 1**, there remains a focus on aggressively reducing modifiable risk factors including elevated LDL-C; this would include the institution of statin therapy either alone or in combination with ezetimibe and/or bile acid sequestrants to achieve LDL-C levels less than 70 mg/dL, or a minimum of 50% reduction in LDL.[70] This recommendation is based on a study of 2769

Table 1
Current and future therapies to lower plasma lipoprotein(a) concentrations

Agent	Status[a]	Mechanism of Action	% ↓ in Lp(a)	Specific for Lp(a)?[b]
Niacin	Approved	Unknown (transcription of *LPA*?)	25	N
Simvastatin	Approved	↑ LDLR	19	N
Atorvastatin	Approved	↑ LDLR	22	N
Mipomersin	Approved (only for homozygous familial hypercholesterolemia)	↓ Translation of apoB mRNA	21–39	N
ASO 144367	Preclinical	↓ Translation of apo(a) mRNA	25 (in Lp[a] Tg mice)	Y
Anacetrapib	Phase III	Unknown	36	N
AMG145	Phase III	Unknown (↑ LDLR?)	30	N
REGN727/ SAR236553	Phase III	Unknown (↑ LDLR?)	30	N
Lomitapibe (AEGR-733)	Phase III	↓ Secretion of apoB-containing lipoproteins	16–19	N
Acetylsalicylic acid	Approved	↓ Transcription of apo(a) mRNA	20	Y
Lipoprotein-apheresis	Approved	Direct removal from plasma	69–73	N
Lp(a)-apheresis	Not available	Direct removal from plasma	73	Y
Tocilizumab	Approved	IL-6 receptor blockade, hence ↓ transcription of apo(a) mRNA	30	Y

[a] Refers to United States; note that no approval has been granted for the indication of elevated Lp(a), specifically.
[b] Refers to lipid profile.
Data from Refs.[25,27,28,42,73–93]

angiography patients wherein risk for major adverse coronary events attributable to Lp(a) was absent in patients with LDL-C less than 70 mg/dL.[71] Another study, in the setting of secondary prevention, found no significant contribution of Lp(a) to risk at LDL-C less than 120 mg/dL.[42] On the other hand, the large JUPITER trial found that a residual risk associated with elevated Lp(a) may persist in the background of low LDL levels resulting from aggressive statin therapy.[44]

It must be emphasized that there have been no randomized clinical trials to date that have specifically addressed the question of whether monitoring Lp(a) concentrations or lowering Lp(a) therapeutically has a clinical benefit. Nonetheless, it seems prudent, given the existing evidence for Lp(a) as a causal risk factor, to measure Lp(a) in specific groups of patients and to tailor their clinical management accordingly.

Some clinicians choose to treat patients with elevated Lp(a) levels using niacin (2 g/d); this may be useful in patients with elevated Lp(a) levels whose LDL concentrations cannot be aggressively lowered or in individuals with Lp(a) levels in excess of 50 mg/dL.[63] However, recent data from the AIM-HIGH trial indicate that niacin treatment did not significantly lower risk for cardiovascular events, despite being able to lower plasma Lp(a) concentrations.[72] Others may choose to include aspirin therapy given that aspirin has been shown to reduce Lp(a) levels and also may mitigate the potential prothrombotic role of Lp(a) in advanced lesions.[73] The latter approach may be of value in patients with existing prothrombotic disorders.[70] In addition to statins, niacin, and aspirin, several drugs in clinical trials or preclinical development have been shown to lower plasma Lp(a) concentrations (**Table 1**).Moreover, LDL-apheresis has been shown to reduce the risk of events attributable to Lp(a)[74,75] and specific Lp(a)-apheresis has been reported to reduce angiographically detectable CHD.[76] Therefore, the coming years may bring novel therapeutic approaches for the patient with elevated plasma Lp(a).

REFERENCES

1. Fless GM, ZumMallen ME, Scanu AM. Physicochemical properties of apolipoprotein(a) and lipoprotein(a−) derived from the dissociation of human plasma lipoprotein (a). J Biol Chem 1986;261:8712–8.
2. Koschinsky ML, Côté GP, Gabel BR, et al. Identification of the cysteine residue in apolipoprotein(a) that mediates extracellular coupling with apolipoprotein B-100. J Biol Chem 1993;268:19819–25.
3. McLean JW, Tomlinson JE, Kuang WJ, et al. cDNA sequence of human apolipoprotein(a) is homologous to plasminogen. Nature 1987;330:132–7.
4. van der Hoek YY, Wittekoek ME, Beisiegel U, et al. The apolipoprotein(a) kringle IV repeats which differ from the major repeat kringle are present in variably-sized isoforms. Hum Mol Genet 1993;2:361–6.
5. Marcovina SM, Albers JJ, Wijsman E, et al. Differences in Lp[a] concentrations and apo[a] polymorphs between black and white Americans. J Lipid Res 1996; 37:2569–85.
6. Lackner C, Cohen JC, Hobbs HH. Molecular definition of the extreme size polymorphism in apolipoprotein(a). Hum Mol Genet 1993;2:933–40.
7. Marcovina SM, Gaur VP, Albers JJ. Biological variability of cholesterol, triglyceride, low- and high-density lipoprotein cholesterol, lipoprotein(a), and apolipoproteins A-I and B. Clin Chem 1994;40:574–8.
8. Utermann G. Genetic architecture and evolution of the lipoprotein(a) trait. Curr Opin Lipidol 1999;10:133–41.

9. Kronenberg F, Utermann G. Lipoprotein(a): resurrected by genetics. J Intern Med 2013;273:6–30.

10. White AL, Guerra B, Lanford RE. Influence of allelic variation on apolipoprotein(a) folding in the endoplasmic reticulum. J Biol Chem 1997;272:5048–55.

11. Brewer HB Jr. Effectiveness of diet and drugs in the treatment of patients with elevated Lp(a) levels. In: Scanu AM, editor. Lipoprotein(a). New York: NY Academic Press, Inc; 1990. p. 211–20.

12. Kamstrup PR, Tybjaerg-Hansen A, Steffensen R, et al. Genetically elevated lipoprotein(a) and increased risk of myocardial infarction. JAMA 2009;301:2331–9.

13. Clarke R, Peden JF, Hopewell JC, et al. Genetic variants associated with Lp(a) lipoprotein level and coronary disease. N Engl J Med 2009;361:2518–28.

14. IBC 50K CAD Consortium. Large-scale gene-centric analysis identifies novel variants for coronary artery disease. PLoS Genet 2011;7:e1002260.

15. Boerwinkle E, Leffert CC, Lin J, et al. Apolipoprotein(a) gene accounts for greater than 90% of the variation in plasma lipoprotein(a) concentrations. J Clin Invest 1992;90:52–60.

16. Dubé JB, Boffa MB, Hegele RA, et al. Lipoprotein(a): more interesting than ever after 50 years. Curr Opin Lipidol 2012;23:133–40.

17. Lanktree MB, Anand SS, Yusuf S, et al. Comprehensive analysis of genomic variation in the LPA locus and its relationship to plasma lipoprotein(a) in South Asians, Chinese, and European Caucasians. Circ Cardiovasc Genet 2010;3:39–46.

18. Luke MM, Kane JP, Liu DM, et al. A polymorphism in the protease-like domain of apolipoprotein(a) is associated with severe coronary artery disease. Arterioscler Thromb Vasc Biol 2007;27:2030–6.

19. Li ZG, Li G, Zhou YL, et al. Lack of association between lipoprotein(a) genetic variants and subsequent cardiovascular events in Chinese Han patients with coronary artery disease after percutaneous coronary intervention. Lipids Health Dis 2013;12:127.

20. Rader DJ, Cain W, Ikewaki K, et al. The inverse association of plasma lipoprotein(a) concentrations with apolipoprotein(a) isoform size is not due to differences in Lp(a) catabolism but to differences in production rate. J Clin Invest 1994;93:2758–63.

21. Cain WJ, Millar JS, Himebauch AS, et al. Lipoprotein [a] is cleared from the plasma primarily by the liver in a process mediated by apolipoprotein [a]. J Lipid Res 2005;46:2681–91.

22. Tam SP, Zhang X, Koschinsky ML. Interaction of a recombinant form of apolipoprotein[a] with human fibroblasts and with the human hepatoma cell line HepG2. J Lipid Res 1996;37:518–33.

23. Rader DJ, Mann WA, Cain W, et al. The low density lipoprotein receptor is not required for normal catabolism of Lp(a) in humans. J Clin Invest 1995;95:1403–8.

24. Gonbert S, Malinsky S, Sposito AC, et al. Atorvastatin lowers lipoprotein(a) but not apolipoprotein(a) fragment levels in hypercholesterolemic subjects at high cardiovascular risk. Atherosclerosis 2002;164:305–11.

25. van Wissen S, Smilde TJ, Trip MD, et al. Long term statin treatment reduces lipoprotein(a) concentrations in heterozygous familial hypercholesterolaemia. Heart 2003;89:893–6.

26. Takagi H, Umemoto T. Atorvastatin decreases lipoprotein(a): a meta-analysis of randomized trials. Int J Cardiol 2012;154:183–6.

27. Desai NR, Kohli P, Giugliano RP, et al. AMG145, a monoclonal antibody against proprotein convertase subtilisin kexin type 9, significantly reduces lipoprotein(a)

in hypercholesterolemic patients receiving statin therapy: an analysis from the LDL-C assessment with proprotein convertase subtilisin kexin type 9 monoclonal antibody inhibition combined with statin therapy (LAPLACE)-thrombolysis in myocardial infarction (TIMI) 57 trial. Circulation 2013;128:962–9.

28. McKenney JM, Koren MJ, Kereiakes DJ, et al. Safety and efficacy of a monoclonal antibody to proprotein convertase subtilisin/kexin type 9 serine protease, SAR236553/REGN727, in patients with primary hypercholesterolemia receiving ongoing stable atorvastatin therapy. J Am Coll Cardiol 2012;59:2344–53.

29. Yang XP, Amar MJ, Vaisman B, et al. Scavenger receptor-BI is a receptor for lipoprotein(a). J Lipid Res 2013;54:2450–7.

30. Boffa MB, Koschinsky ML. Update on lipoprotein(a) as a cardiovascular risk factor and mediator. Curr Atheroscler Rep 2013;15:360.

31. Anglés-Cano E, de la Peña Díaz A, Loyau S. Inhibition of fibrinolysis by lipoprotein(a). Ann N Y Acad Sci 2001;936:261–75.

32. Seimon TA, Nadolski MJ, Liao X, et al. Atherogenic lipids and lipoproteins trigger CD36-TLR2-dependent apoptosis in macrophages undergoing endoplasmic reticulum stress. Cell Metab 2010;12:467–82.

33. Cho T, Jung Y, Koschinsky ML. Apolipoprotein(a), through its strong lysine-binding site in KIV(10'), mediates increased endothelial cell contraction and permeability via a Rho/Rho kinase/MYPT1-dependent pathway. J Biol Chem 2008;283:30503–12.

34. Cho T, Romagnuolo R, Scipione C, et al. Apolipoprotein(a) stimulates nuclear translocation of β-catenin: a novel pathogenic mechanism for lipoprotein(a). Mol Biol Cell 2013;24:210–21.

35. Tsimikas S, Mallat Z, Talmud PJ, et al. Oxidation-specific biomarkers, lipoprotein(a), and risk of fatal and nonfatal coronary events. J Am Coll Cardiol 2010; 56:946–55.

36. Tsimikas S, Bergmark C, Beyer RW, et al. Temporal increases in plasma markers of oxidized low-density lipoprotein strongly reflect the presence of acute coronary syndromes. J Am Coll Cardiol 2003;41:360–70.

37. Bergmark C, Dewan A, Orsoni A, et al. A novel function of lipoprotein [a] as a preferential carrier of oxidized phospholipids in human plasma. J Lipid Res 2008;49:2230–9.

38. Leibundgut G, Scipione C, Yin H, et al. Determinants of binding of oxidized phospholipids on apolipoprotein (a) and lipoprotein (a). J Lipid Res 2013;54: 2815–30.

39. Hughes SD, Lou XJ, Ighani S, et al. Lipoprotein(a) vascular accumulation in mice. In vivo analysis of the role of lysine binding sites using recombinant adenovirus. J Clin Invest 1997;100:1493–500.

40. Deshmane SL, Kremlev S, Amini S, et al. Monocyte chemoattractant protein-1 (MCP-1): an overview. J Interferon Cytokine Res 2009;29:313–26.

41. Wiesner P, Tafelmeier M, Chittka D, et al. MCP-1 binds to oxidized LDL and is carried by lipoprotein(a) in human plasma. J Lipid Res 2013;54:1877–83.

42. O'Donoghue ML, Morrow DA, Tsimikas S, et al. Lipoprotein(a) for risk assessment in patients with established coronary artery disease. J Am Coll Cardiol 2014;63:520–7.

43. Nestel PJ, Barnes EH, Tonkin AM, et al. Plasma lipoprotein(a) concentration predicts future coronary and cardiovascular events in patients with stable coronary heart disease. Arterioscler Thromb Vasc Biol 2013;33:2902–8.

44. Khera AV, Everett BM, Caulfield MP, et al. Lipoprotein(a) concentrations, rosuvastatin therapy, and residual vascular risk: an analysis from the JUPITER trial

(justification for the use of statins in prevention: an intervention trial evaluating rosuvastatin). Circulation 2014;129:635–42.

45. Thanassoulis G, Campbell CY, Owens DS, et al. Genetic associations with valvular calcification and aortic stenosis. N Engl J Med 2013;368:503–12.

46. Kamstrup PR, Tybjærg-Hansen A, Nordestgaard BG. Elevated lipoprotein(a) and risk of aortic valve stenosis in the general population. J Am Coll Cardiol 2014;63:470–7.

47. Kamstrup PR, Tybjærg-Hansen A, Nordestgaard BG. Genetic evidence that lipoprotein(a) associates with atherosclerotic stenosis rather than venous thrombosis. Arterioscler Thromb Vasc Biol 2012;32:1732–41.

48. Danik JS, Buring JE, Chasman DI, et al. Lipoprotein(a), polymorphisms in the LPA gene, and incident venous thromboembolism among 21483 women. J Thromb Haemost 2013;11:205–8.

49. Helgadottir A, Gretarsdottir S, Thorleifsson G, et al. Apolipoprotein(a) genetic sequence variants associated with systemic atherosclerosis and coronary atherosclerotic burden but not with venous thromboembolism. J Am Coll Cardiol 2012;60:722–9.

50. Undas A, Cieśla-Dul M, Drążkiewicz T, et al. Altered fibrin clot properties are associated with residual vein obstruction: effects of lipoprotein(a) and apolipoprotein(a) isoform. Thromb Res 2012;130:e184–7.

51. Rowland CM, Pullinger CR, Luke MM, et al. Lipoprotein (a), LPA Ile4399Met, and fibrin clot properties. Thromb Res 2014;133:863–7.

52. Kardys I, Oemrawsingh RM, Kay IP, et al. Lipoprotein(a), interleukin-10, C-reactive protein, and 8-year outcome after percutaneous coronary intervention. Clin Cardiol 2012;35:482–9.

53. Greif M, Arnoldt T, von Ziegler F, et al. Lipoprotein (a) is independently correlated with coronary artery calcification. Eur J Intern Med 2013;24:75–9.

54. Sung KC, Wild SH, Byrne CD. Lipoprotein (a), metabolic syndrome and coronary calcium score in a large occupational cohort. Nutr Metab Cardiovasc Dis 2013;23:1239–46.

55. Sharma A, Kasim M, Joshi PH, et al. Abnormal lipoprotein(a) levels predict coronary artery calcification in Southeast Asians but not in Caucasians: use of noninvasive imaging for evaluation of an emerging risk factor. J Cardiovasc Transl Res 2011;4:470–6.

56. Erbel R, Lehmann N, Churzidse S, et al. Gender-specific association of coronary artery calcium and lipoprotein parameters: the Heinz Nixdorf recall study. Atherosclerosis 2013;229:531–40.

57. Qasim AN, Martin SS, Mehta NN, et al. Lipoprotein(a) is strongly associated with coronary artery calcification in type-2 diabetic women. Int J Cardiol 2011;150:17–21.

58. Brown WV, Ballantyne CM, Jones PH, et al. Management of Lp(a). J Clin Lipidol 2010;4:240–7.

59. Hopewell JC, Seedorf U, Farrall M, et al. Impact of lipoprotein(a) levels and apolipoprotein(a) isoform size on risk of coronary heart disease. J Intern Med 2013;276(3):260–8. http://dx.doi.org/10.1111/joim.12187.

60. Anderson TJ, Grégoire J, Hegele RA, et al. 2012 update of the Canadian Cardiovascular Society guidelines for the diagnosis and treatment of dyslipidemia for the prevention of cardiovascular disease in the adult. Can J Cardiol 2013;29:151–67.

61. Virani SS, Brautbar A, Davis BC, et al. Associations between lipoprotein(a) levels and cardiovascular outcomes in black and white subjects: the atherosclerosis risk in communities (ARIC) study. Circulation 2012;125:241–9.

62. Kamstrup PR, Tybjærg-Hansen A, Nordestgaard BG. Extreme lipoprotein(a) levels and improved cardiovascular risk prediction. J Am Coll Cardiol 2013; 61:1146–56.

63. Nordestgaard BG, Chapman MJ, Ray K, et al. Lipoprotein(a) as a cardiovascular risk factor: current status. Eur Heart J 2010;31:2844–53.

64. Greenland P, Alpert JS, Beller GA, et al. American College of Cardiology Foundation; American Heart Association. 2010 ACCF/AHA guideline for assessment of cardiovascular risk in asymptomatic adults. J Am Coll Cardiol 2010;56:e50–103.

65. Kostner KM, März W, Kostner GM. When should we measure lipoprotein (a)? Eur Heart J 2013;34:3268–76.

66. Marcovina SM, Koschinsky ML, Albers JJ, et al. Report of the National Heart, Lung, and Blood Institute workshop on lipoprotein(a) and cardiovascular disease: recent advances and future directions. Clin Chem 2003;49:1785–96.

67. Seman LJ, DeLuca C, Jenner JL, et al. Lipoprotein(a)-cholesterol and coronary heart disease in the Framingham heart study. Clin Chem 1999;45:1039–46.

68. Konerman M, Kulkarni K, Toth PP, et al. Lipoprotein(a) particle concentration and lipoprotein(a) cholesterol assays yield discordant classification of patients into four physiologically discrete groups. J Clin Lipidol 2012;6:368–73.

69. Lamon-Fava S, Marcovina SM, Albers JJ, et al. Lipoprotein(a) levels, apo(a) isoform size, and coronary heart disease risk in the Framingham Offspring Study. J Lipid Res 2011;52:1181–7.

70. Jacobson TA. Lipoprotein(a), cardiovascular disease, and contemporary management. Mayo Clin Proc 2013;88:1294–311.

71. Nicholls SJ, Tang WH, Scoffone H, et al. Lipoprotein(a) levels and long-term cardiovascular risk in the contemporary era of statin therapy. J Lipid Res 2010;51: 3055–61.

72. Albers JJ, Slee A, O'Brien KD, et al. Relationship of apolipoproteins A-1 and B, and lipoprotein(a) to cardiovascular outcomes: the AIM-HIGH trial (atherothrombosis intervention in metabolic syndrome with low HDL/high triglyceride and impact on global health outcomes). J Am Coll Cardiol 2013;62:1575–9.

73. Chasman DI, Shiffman D, Zee RY, et al. Polymorphism in the apolipoprotein(a) gene, plasma lipoprotein(a), cardiovascular disease, and low-dose aspirin therapy. Atherosclerosis 2009;203:371–6.

74. Jaeger BR, Richter Y, Nagel D, et al. Longitudinal cohort study on the effectiveness of lipid apheresis treatment to reduce high lipoprotein(a) levels and prevent major adverse coronary events. Nat Clin Pract Cardiovasc Med 2009;6: 229–39.

75. Leebmann J, Roeseler E, Julius U, et al. Lipoprotein apheresis in patients with maximally tolerated lipid-lowering therapy, lipoprotein(a)-hyperlipoproteinemia, and progressive cardiovascular disease: prospective observational multicenter study. Circulation 2013;128:2567–76.

76. Safarova MS, Ezhov MV, Afanasieva OI, et al. Effect of specific lipoprotein(a) apheresis on coronary atherosclerosis regression assessed by quantitative coronary angiography. Atheroscler Suppl 2013;14:93–9.

77. Boden WE, Probstfield JL, Anderson T, et al. Niacin in patients with low HDL cholesterol levels receiving intensive statin therapy. N Engl J Med 2011;365: 2255–67.

78. Besseling J, Hovingh GK, Stroes ES. Antisense oligonucleotides in the treatment of lipid disorders: pitfalls and promises. Neth J Med 2013;71:118–22.

79. Raal FJ, Santos RD, Blom DJ, et al. Mipomersen, an apolipoprotein B synthesis inhibitor, for lowering of LDL cholesterol concentrations in patients with

homozygous familial hypercholesterolaemia: a randomised, double-blind, placebo-controlled trial. Lancet 2010;375:998–1006.

80. Stein EA, Dufour R, Gagne C, et al. Apolipoprotein B synthesis inhibition with mipomersen in heterozygous familial hypercholesterolemia: results of a randomized, double-blind, placebo-controlled trial to assess efficacy and safety as add-on therapy in patients with coronary artery disease. Circulation 2012;126: 2283–92.

81. McGowan MP, Tardif JC, Ceska R, et al. Randomized, placebo-controlled trial of mipomersen in patients with severe hypercholesterolemia receiving maximally tolerated lipid-lowering therapy. PLoS One 2012;7:e49006.

82. Thomas GS, Cromwell WC, Ali S, et al. Mipomersen, an apolipoprotein B synthesis inhibitor, reduces atherogenic lipoproteins in patients with severe hypercholesterolemia at high cardiovascular risk: a randomized, double-blind, placebo-controlled trial. J Am Coll Cardiol 2013;62:2178–84.

83. Visser ME, Wagener G, Baker BF, et al. Mipomersen, an apolipoprotein B synthesis inhibitor, lowers low-density lipoprotein cholesterol in high-risk statin-intolerant patients: a randomized, double-blind, placebo-controlled trial. Eur Heart J 2012;33:1142–9.

84. Merki E, Graham M, Taleb A, et al. Antisense oligonucleotide lowers plasma levels of apolipoprotein (a) and lipoprotein (a) in transgenic mice. J Am Coll Cardiol 2011;57:1611–21.

85. Cannon CP, Shah S, Dansky HM, et al. Safety of anacetrapib in patients with or at high risk for coronary heart disease. N Engl J Med 2010;363:2406–15.

86. Dias CS, Shaywitz AJ, Wasserman SM, et al. Effects of AMG 145 on low-density lipoprotein cholesterol levels: results from 2 randomized, double-blind, placebo-controlled, ascending-dose phase 1 studies in healthy volunteers and hypercholesterolemic subjects on statins. J Am Coll Cardiol 2012;60:1888–98.

87. Raal F, Scott R, Somaratne R, et al. Low-density lipoprotein cholesterol-lowering effects of AMG 145, a monoclonal antibody to proprotein convertase subtilisin/kexin type 9 serine protease in patients with heterozygous familial hypercholesterolemia: the reduction of LDL-C with PCSK9 Inhibition in heterozygous familial hypercholesterolemia disorder (RUTHERFORD) randomized trial. Circulation 2012;126:2408–17.

88. Sullivan D, Olsson AG, Scott R, et al. Effect of a monoclonal antibody to PCSK9 on low-density lipoprotein cholesterol levels in statin-intolerant patients: the GAUSS randomized trial. JAMA 2012;308:2497–506.

89. Roth EM, McKenney JM, Hanotin C, et al. Atorvastatin with or without an antibody to PCSK9 in primary hypercholesterolemia. N Engl J Med 2012;367: 1891–900.

90. Cuchel M, Bloedon LT, Szapary PO, et al. Inhibition of microsomal triglyceride transfer protein in familial hypercholesterolemia. N Engl J Med 2007;356:148–56.

91. Cuchel M, Meagher EA, du Toit Theron H, et al. Efficacy and safety of a microsomal triglyceride transfer protein inhibitor in patients with homozygous familial hypercholesterolaemia: a single-arm, open-label, phase 3 study. Lancet 2013; 381:40–6.

92. Samaha FF, McKenney J, Bloedon LT, et al. Inhibition of microsomal triglyceride transfer protein alone or with ezetimibe in patients with moderate hypercholesterolemia. Nat Clin Pract Cardiovasc Med 2008;5:497–505.

93. Schultz O, Oberhauser F, Saech J, et al. Effects of inhibition of interleukin-6 signalling on insulin sensitivity and lipoprotein (a) levels in human subjects with rheumatoid diseases. PLoS One 2010;5:e14328.

Recent Findings of Studies on the Mediterranean Diet

What are the Implications for Current Dietary Recommendations?

Chesney K. Richter, BS, PhD(c), Ann C. Skulas-Ray, PhD,
Penny M. Kris-Etherton, PhD, RD*

KEYWORDS

- Mediterranean diet • Dietary recommendations • Dietary patterns
- Cardiovascular disease • Clinical trials

KEY POINTS

- Current dietary guidelines (eg, Dietary Guidelines for Americans 2010 and 2013 American Heart Association/American College of Cardiology Guideline on Lifestyle Management to Reduce Cardiovascular Risk) recommend a dietary pattern approach for reducing chronic disease risk.
- The Dietary Approaches to Stop Hypertension (DASH) diet and United States Department of Agriculture Food Patterns are the primary dietary patterns recommended in the current guidelines.
- There is a robust evidence base demonstrating that the Mediterranean dietary pattern also can reduce the risk of many chronic diseases, including cardiovascular disease (CVD).
- A Mediterranean-style diet is consistent with most dietary guidelines issued recently, and with modifications to reduce sodium and saturated fat, can meet current recommendations.
- Including the Mediterranean diet as one of the recommended evidence-based dietary patterns may help individuals achieve better long-term dietary adherence and, thus, sustain optimal reductions in CVD risk.

INTRODUCTION: DIETARY GUIDELINES AND RECOMMENDED DIETARY PATTERNS

A healthy diet has long been a cornerstone for the prevention and treatment of cardiovascular disease (CVD). The American Heart Association (AHA) first published dietary recommendations for CVD risk reduction in 1957 and regularly updates them as new

The authors have nothing to disclose.
Department of Nutritional Sciences, The Pennsylvania State University, 110 Chandlee Laboratory, University Park, PA 16802, USA
* Corresponding author.
E-mail address: pmk3@psu.edu

Endocrinol Metab Clin N Am 43 (2014) 963–980
http://dx.doi.org/10.1016/j.ecl.2014.08.003
0889-8529/14/$ – see front matter © 2014 Elsevier Inc. All rights reserved.

science emerges.[1] The United States Department of Agriculture (USDA) and the Department of Health and Human Services also continually update diet and lifestyle recommendations to reduce chronic disease risk. Traditionally, dietary recommendations have targeted macronutrient levels, particularly the type and amount of dietary fat. However, the most recent dietary guidelines (eg, Dietary Guidelines for Americans [DGA] 2010 and 2013 American Heart Association/American College of Cardiology [AHA/ACC] Guideline on Lifestyle Management to Reduce Cardiovascular Risk) have shifted toward a more food-based dietary pattern approach for preventing CVD and reducing CVD risk factors.[2,3] This approach integrates all nutrient recommendations and targets multiple CVD risk factors, as well as many other chronic diseases, with the aim of producing greater health benefits.

There is a strong evidence base demonstrating the efficacy of multiple dietary patterns in reducing CVD risk factors, morbidity, and mortality. The Dietary Approaches to Stop Hypertension (DASH) diet,[4,5] USDA Food Patterns,[2] and Mediterranean-type diets[6–8] are discussed in both the Dietary Guidelines for Americans 2010 and the 2013 AHA/ACC Guideline on Lifestyle Management; however, there is an emphasis on implementing the DASH Diet and USDA Food Patterns to meet dietary targets (**Table 1**). These 3 dietary patterns share many common features, including higher intake of plant-based foods and lean protein instead of foods that contain higher amounts of saturated fat. **Fig. 1** summarizes the key recommendations of these dietary patterns and illustrates their commonalities (eg, an emphasis on "nutrient-dense foods" such as vegetables, fruits, whole grains, seafood, eggs, low-fat dairy, nuts, lean meats, and poultry while limiting saturated fat, trans fat, added sugars, and refined grains[2]) and unique features, such as emphasis on salt restriction or higher intake of omega-3 fatty acids. Derivatives of the DASH dietary patterns in which 10% of total daily energy from carbohydrates is replaced with either protein or unsaturated fat were shown to be effective in lowering CVD risk factors in the OmniHeart Study.[9] Thus, macronutrient variations of the DASH dietary pattern provide additional options that can be implemented to reduce CVD risk.

The availability of different evidence-based dietary patterns provides greater flexibility in accommodating personal preferences, which is crucial for achieving the long-term adherence required for significant CVD risk reduction. These whole food approaches benefit multiple traditional CVD risk factors, including lipids and lipoproteins, blood pressure, insulin sensitivity, and body weight, in addition to emerging risk factors.[10–12] Healthy dietary patterns provide multiple cardioprotective bioactives, such as omega-3 fatty acids and plant-derived antioxidants, and, therefore, confer additional cardiovascular benefits beyond the recommended macronutrient profile.

Evidence-based dietary patterns are highlighted in the most recent dietary guidelines for reducing the risk of CVD and other chronic diseases (eg, DGA 2010 and 2013 AHA/ACC Lifestyle Guideline),[2,3] which encourage nutrient-dense foods, particularly those high in dietary fiber, vitamin D, calcium, and potassium. **Table 1** summarizes the key messages from these guidelines. The DASH diet is the primary dietary pattern recommended by the 2013 AHA/ACC Guideline for the reduction of low-density lipoprotein (LDL) cholesterol (LDL-C) and blood pressure, two major risk factors for CVD.[3] This dietary pattern is relatively low in total fat (27%–28% of total calories), saturated fat ($\sim$6% of total calories), and sodium (1500 mg/day). The AHA/ACC Guideline also recommends a Mediterranean dietary pattern and variations in the DASH dietary pattern that are higher in total fat (ie, largely from unsaturated fat) and total protein (ie, with an emphasis on plant protein). However, the strength of evidence for a Mediterranean dietary pattern on lowering blood pressure and LDL-C was deemed "low" according to the AHA/ACC grading methodology. Thus, the emphasis

Table 1
Key recommendations from the current dietary guidelines to reduce the risk of cardiovascular disease (CVD)

	Total Fat (% of Calories)	Saturated Fat (% of Calories)	Trans Fat	Cholesterol	Sodium	Alcohol	Recommended Dietary Patterns[a]	Foods to Emphasize	Foods to Limit
Dietary Guidelines for Americans (DGA) 2010	20–35	*Replace with MUFAs and PUFAs* <10	Keep consumption as low as possible	<300 mg/d	<2300 mg/d <1500 mg/d if 51+ years old, African American, and/or have *hypertension, diabetes, or chronic kidney disease*	In moderation 1 drink/d for women, 2/d for men	DASH diet USDA Food Patterns	Vegetables and fruits, whole grains, fat-free or low-fat milk/milk products, seafood, lean meat and poultry, eggs, beans, soy, unsalted nuts and seeds. Use oils to replace solid fats. Foods that provide more potassium, fiber, calcium, and vitamin D	Refined grains, solid fats, and added sugars
2013 AHA/ACC Guideline on Lifestyle Management to Reduce Cardiovascular Risk	—[b]	5–6	Reduce % of calories from trans fat	—[c]	Reduce sodium intake by at least 1000 mg/d *No more than 2400 mg/d; further reduction to 1500 mg/d is desirable*	—[d]	DASH diet USDA Food Patterns	Vegetables, fruits, whole grains, low-fat dairy products, poultry, fish, legumes, nontropical vegetable oils and nuts	Sweets, sugar-sweetened beverages, red meats

Abbreviations: AHA/ACC, American Heart Association/American College of Cardiology; DASH, Dietary Approaches to Stop Hypertension; MUFA, monounsaturated fatty acid; PUFA, polyunsaturated fatty acid; USDA, United States Department of Agriculture.

[a] Both the DGA 2010 and 2013 AHA/ACC Guideline discuss research on the Mediterranean dietary pattern but emphasize the DASH diet and USDA Food Patterns for meeting specific recommendations.
[b] Not specified. The DASH diet was deemed to have the strongest evidence base by the 2013 AHA/ACC Work Group and contains 26%–27% total fat.
[c] Deemed to have insufficient evidence for lowering low-density lipoprotein cholesterol.
[d] Not included in the scope of the Guideline.

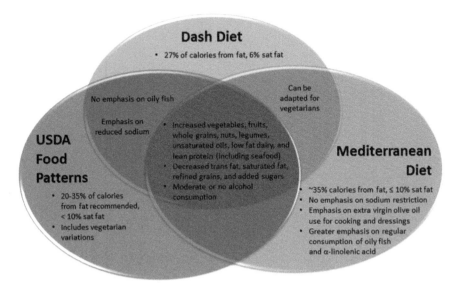

Fig. 1. Commonalities and unique features of the DASH diet, USDA food patterns, and Mediterranean diet.

of the AHA/ACC Guideline has been on the DASH dietary pattern, with its "strong" evidence for benefiting lipids/lipoproteins and improving blood pressure. According to the 2013 AHA/ACC Evidence Statements, when compared with the average American diet the DASH dietary pattern lowers LDL-C by 11 mg/dL, systolic blood pressure (SBP) by 5 to 6 mm Hg, and diastolic blood pressure (DBP) by 3 mm Hg.[3] However, the scope of the AHA/ACC Guideline focused primarily on modifiable CVD risk factors (eg, lipids/lipoproteins and blood pressure) rather than cardiovascular events and did not review the evidence for morbidity and mortality in regard to dietary patterns. As such, the 2013 AHA/ACC Guideline does not incorporate the most recent results from PREDIMED,[3] the only large-scale randomized controlled trial that has evaluated the effect of a Mediterranean diet intervention on the primary prevention of CVD.

There is growing evidence that the Mediterranean dietary pattern decreases risk factors for many chronic diseases, including CVD. Both epidemiologic studies and controlled clinical trials demonstrate that a Mediterranean dietary pattern decreases the risk of cardiovascular events and major CVD risk factors. This article summarizes recent clinical trial research on the cardiovascular benefits of a Mediterranean dietary pattern. This evidence provides the basis for recommending a Mediterranean dietary pattern in clinical practice to reduce the risk of CVD.

MEDITERRANEAN DIET: OVERVIEW AND EVIDENCE BASE

The Mediterranean dietary pattern represents the food habits and cultural practices of the countries that surround the Mediterranean Sea.[13] Although there are country-specific variations in the foods consumed, which have also changed over time, there are commonalities in food groups and their frequency of consumption. Although the dietary pattern referred to as "The" Mediterranean diet does not entirely replicate the intake of any one region in particular, it most closely resembles the characteristics of the diet traditionally consumed in Crete, as described by Ancel Keys in 1970.[14] The characteristics of this dietary pattern are depicted in **Fig. 2**. Typically, the

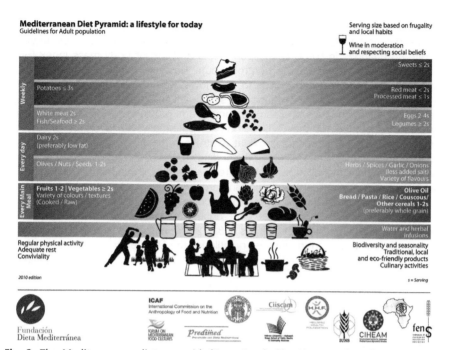

Fig. 2. The Mediterranean diet pyramid. (*From* Fundación Dieta Mediterránea. The New Mediterranean Diet Pyramid. 2010. Available at: http://dietamediterranea.com/en/the-fdm-presents-the-new-mediterranean-diet-pyramid/. Accessed June 28, 2014.)

recommended Mediterranean dietary pattern is moderate in total fat (32%–35% of total calories), relatively low in saturated fat (9%–10% of total calories), high in fiber (27–37 g/d), and high in monounsaturated and polyunsaturated fatty acids, with an emphasis on omega-3 fatty acids. It emphasizes fresh fruits, root and green vegetables, grains (mostly whole), legumes, fatty fish rich in omega-3 fatty acids, nuts, seeds, and olive oil in place of butter or other animal-based fats. Lower-fat or fat-free dairy products are consumed daily; fish, poultry, and eggs are consumed in low to moderate amounts; and red meat and sweets are limited. Wine is also consumed in low to moderate amounts in non-Islamic countries. This dietary pattern also reflects the Mediterranean way of life, which includes regular physical activity, adequate rest, and engaging social/family relationships.

Great interest in the Mediterranean diet was generated in the 1980s by reports from The Seven Countries Study, which found that the 15-year mortality rate from CVD in the Mediterranean region of Southern Europe was substantially lower than in Northern Europe and the United States.[15] This finding was hypothesized to be due to the dietary habits of these populations, as regions with the highest CVD mortality also had greater saturated fat intake and higher serum cholesterol levels. Subsequently, the Lyon Diet Heart Study[16] was designed to test the effects of a Mediterranean diet on secondary prevention of myocardial infarction (MI), relative to a prudent Western-style diet. Subjects were randomized to consume a prudent Western-style diet or a Mediterranean-style diet lower in saturated fat and higher in α-linolenic acid from a canola oil–based margarine for 104 weeks. Subjects in the Mediterranean-style diet group were advised to consume more bread, root vegetables, green vegetables, and fish; less meat; fruit every day; and replace butter and cream with margarine supplied by the study. The

Mediterranean-style diet treatment group had a markedly lower prevalence of cardiac death and nonfatal MI, fewer major secondary events, and decreased hospitalizations despite no changes in blood lipids/lipoproteins and similar body mass index (BMI) and blood pressure versus the control group. Because subjects consuming the Mediterranean-style diet had a 50% to 70% lower risk of recurrent cardiac events, the study was stopped early because of a significant CVD benefit.[16] It has been suggested that the abundance of bioactive compounds provided by the Mediterranean-style diet accounted for the CVD outcomes, potentially via favorable effects on vascular function, arrhythmia, and oxidative stress.

Subsequent studies have validated the findings of the Lyon Diet Heart Study. Meta-analyses have consistently reported that greater adherence to a Mediterranean diet is associated with a significant reduction in cardiovascular mortality and total mortality.[17-19] A further meta-analysis of cohort studies by Mente and colleagues[20] also found strong evidence that greater adherence to a Mediterranean dietary pattern was protective against CVD. An analysis of 81,722 women in the Nurses' Health Study also found that women in the highest quintile for the Mediterranean diet score (high intake of vegetables, fruits, nuts, whole grains, legumes, fish; ratio of monounsaturated fatty acids to saturated fatty acids; moderate intake of alcohol; and low intake of red and processed meat), experienced a 40% reduction in sudden cardiac death relative to the women consuming diets least reflective of this dietary pattern.[21] In addition, a meta-analysis of 50 prospective studies and clinical trials reported that greater adherence to the Mediterranean diet reduced the risk of metabolic syndrome and improved specific metabolic syndrome criteria (ie, waist circumference, high-density lipoprotein cholesterol [HDL-C] triglycerides [TG], SBP and DBP, and glucose).[22] The most recent systematic reviews of cross-sectional, prospective cohort, and intervention studies have demonstrated further the favorable effects of a Mediterranean-style dietary pattern,[23] in terms of both a reduction in cardiovascular events[24] and improvements in many traditional CVD risk factors, including blood lipids/lipoproteins, body weight and BMI, SBP and DBP, fasting glucose and insulin resistance, and C-reactive protein.[25,26]

In addition to the epidemiologic evidence, numerous short-term intervention trials have evaluated the effects of a Mediterranean-style diet on CVD risk factors (**Table 2**). These trials provide additional evidence for the beneficial effects of a Mediterranean-style dietary pattern on the following CVD risk factors: plasma lipid/lipoprotein profiles,[27-31] apolipoproteins,[28] body weight/composition,[29,32,33] oxidative stress,[34] glycemic response,[27,29,32,33] inflammatory markers,[28,29] vascular function,[29,35-38] and criteria for metabolic syndrome.[29] However, some studies have not reported CVD benefits of a Mediterranean-style dietary pattern.[6,7,39-41] This finding may reflect differences in study design, duration, and type of control/comparator diets evaluated. There also is a lack of morbidity and mortality data, which affects the strength of the evidence.

The Lyon Diet Heart Study was the only clinical trial evaluating the effect of a Mediterranean-style diet on cardiovascular morbidity and mortality until Prevención con Dieta Mediterránea (PREDIMED) began in 2003. PREDIMED, a multicenter clinical trial, evaluated the efficacy of a Mediterranean diet on the primary prevention of CVD. Participants were 55 to 80 years of age with type 2 diabetes or with 3 or more major CVD risk factors (hypertension, hypercholesterolemia, family history of heart disease, tobacco use, or overweight/obesity) and randomized to: (1) a low(er)-fat diet, (2) a Mediterranean diet with extra-virgin olive oil (EVOO) (1 L/wk/family; 50 g/d per participant), or (3) a Mediterranean diet with tree nuts (30 g/d: 15 g walnuts, 7.5 g hazelnuts, 7.5 g almonds).[8,42] After 3 months, subjects in both Mediterranean diet groups had

Table 2
Studies evaluating the effect of a Mediterranean-style diet intervention on cardiovascular disease (CVD) risk factors

Authors,[Ref.] Year	Location of Study	Design	Duration	Population	Intervention	Control or Comparator Diet	Main Findings[a]
Elhayany et al,[27] 2010	Israel	Parallel	1 y	Overweight patients with T2DM (n = 259)	Traditional Mediterranean diet (TM)	Low-CHO Mediterranean (LCM) diet and 2003 American Diabetes Association (ADA) diet	Greater reduction in TG with both LCM and TM Only LCM increased HDL-C and resulted in greater HbA1c reduction
Esposito et al,[32] 2009	Italy	Parallel	4 y	Overweight subjects with newly diagnosed T2DM (n = 215)	Mediterranean-style diet (<50% daily calories from CHO)	Low-fat diet (<30% daily calories from fat)	Delayed need for antihyperglycemic drug therapy, and greater decreases in body weight, glycemic control, and coronary risk measures
Tuttle et al,[39] 2008	USA	Parallel	46 mo	Patients with history of MI (n = 101)	Mediterranean-style dietary counseling	Low-fat diet comparator and usual-care control	No significant difference in survival between Mediterranean and low-fat groups (both interventions improved outcomes relative to usual-care control)
Michalsen et al,[40] 2006	Germany	Parallel	1 y	Patients with CAD (n = 101, 80% treated with statins)	100 h of education about Mediterranean diet	Written advice-only	No changes in markers of inflammation and metabolic risk factors

(continued on next page)

Table 2
(continued)

Authors,[Ref.] Year	Location of Study	Design	Duration	Population	Intervention	Control or Comparator Diet	Main Findings[a]
Stachowska et al,[34] 2005	Poland	Parallel	6 mo	Kidney graft recipients (n = 37)	Mediterranean diet	Low-fat diet	Greater decreases in oxidative stress
Vincent-Baudry et al,[7] 2005	France	Parallel	3 mo	Individuals with moderate CVD risk (≥1 risk factor) (n = 212)	Mediterranean-style diet (35%–38% total fat)	AHA-type diet (30% total fat)	No significant differences between groups; Trend for greater reduction in TC and LDL-C; Predicted 9% CVD risk reduction with low-fat diet vs 15% CVD risk reduction with MD
Bravo-Herrera et al,[28] 2004	Spain	Crossover	3 mo	Healthy participants (n = 41)	Mediterranean diet	Low-fat high-CHO diet and SFA-enriched diet	Improved all outcomes except HDL-C relative to high-fat diet; Reduced HDL-C and apo A-I less than low-fat diet
Esposito et al,[29] 2004	Italy	Parallel	2 y	Individuals with metabolic syndrome (n = 180)	Mediterranean diet	Prudent Western diet	Greater improvements in all outcomes (body weight, BMI, waist circumference, CRP, IL-6, IL-7, IL-18, glucose, HOMA-IR, TC, TG, HDL-C, SBP and DBP, endothelial function, features of metabolic syndrome)

Study	Country	Design	Duration	Participants	MUFA diet (40% total fat)	CHO diet (28% total fat)	Outcomes
Rodriguez-Villar et al,[31] 2004	Spain	Crossover	6 wk	Patients with T2DM (n = 22)			Greater reductions in VLDL-C and VLDL-TG
Ros et al,[54] 2004	Spain	Crossover	4 wk	Participants with hypercholesterolemia (n = 21)	Mediterranean diet	Similar diet with walnuts (replaced 32% of energy from MUFAs)	Walnut diet produced greater reduction in TC, LDL-C, VCAM-1, and improved endothelium-dependent vasodilation
Sondergaard et al,[35] 2003	Denmark	Parallel	1 y	Patients with IHD and hypercholesterolemia (n = 131)	Mediterranean dietary advice (both groups received 40 mg Fluvastatin)	Usual diet	Improved endothelial function
Toobert et al,[33] 2003	USA	Parallel	6 mo	Postmenopausal women with T2DM (n = 279)	Mediterranean Lifestyle Program	Usual diet	Greater improvements in HbA1c, BMI, plasma fatty acids, and quality of life
Singh et al,[36] 2002	UK	Parallel	6 wk	Healthy participants (n = 54)	Mediterranean diet	1 g/d vitamin C or placebo	Improved endothelium-dependent and endothelium-independent dilation
Fuentes et al,[37] 2001	Spain	Crossover	4 wk	Men with hypercholesterolemia (n = 22)	Mediterranean diet	Low-fat NCEP-1 diet following high-fat high-SFA run-in	Improved flow-mediated dilation
Mezzano et al,[55] 2001	Chile	Parallel	3 mo	Healthy participants (n = 42)	Mediterranean diet (with wine added after second month)	High-fat diet	Reduced plasma fibrinogen, factor VIIc, and factor VIIIc; and higher protein S Red wine consumption enhanced improvements

(continued on next page)

Table 2
(continued)

Authors,[Ref.] Year	Location of Study	Design	Duration	Population	Intervention	Control or Comparator Diet	Main Findings[a]
Perez-Jimenez et al,[41] 2001	Spain	Crossover	4 wk	Healthy participants (n = 59)	Mediterranean diet (following high-fat high-SFA baseline diet)	High-CHO diet	No differences in outcomes
Zambon et al,[56] 2000	Spain	Crossover	6 wk	Patients with hypercholesterolemia (n = 49)	Mediterranean diet	Similar diet with walnuts (replaced 35% MUFAs)	Walnut diet produced greater reductions in TC, LDL-C, lipoprotein a, LDL:HDL ratio, and apolipoprotein B
de Lorgeril et al,[6] 1999	France	Parallel	46 mo	Men and women with previous MI	Mediterranean-style diet with high-ALA margarine provided	Prudent AHA diet	No significant differences in traditional CVD risk factors (TC, LDL-C, and blood pressure)
Strazzullo et al,[38] 1986	Italy	Sequential	6 wk	Healthy participants (n = 57)	Mediterranean diet	High-fat Western diet	Lower SBP
Ferro-Luzzi et al,[30] 1984	Italy	Sequential	6 wk	Healthy participants (n = 48)	Mediterranean diet	High-fat Western diet	Lower LDL-C and TC

Abbreviations: AHA, American Heart Association; ALA, α-linolenic acid; apo, apolipoprotein; BMI, body mass index; CAD, coronary artery disease; CHO, carbohydrate; CRP, C-reactive protein; DBP, diastolic blood pressure; HbA1c, hemoglobin A1c; HDL, high-density lipoprotein; HDL-C, high-density lipoprotein cholesterol; HOMA-IR, homeostatic model assessment of insulin resistance; IHD, ischemic heart disease; IL, interleukin; LDL, low-density lipoprotein; LDL-C, low-density lipoprotein cholesterol; MI, myocardial infarction; NCEP, National Cholesterol Education Program; SBP, systolic blood pressure; SFA, saturated fatty acid; TC, total cholesterol; TG, triglycerides; T2DM, type 2 diabetes mellitus; VCAM, vascular cell adhesion molecule; VLDL, very low-density lipoprotein; VLDL-C, very low-density lipoprotein cholesterol.

[a] Mediterranean-style intervention diet compared to control and/or comparator diet(s).

Data from Refs.[6,7,27–41,54–56]

Table 3
Studies evaluating the effect of a Mediterranean-style diet intervention on cardiovascular events and mortality

Trial	Reference	Location of Study	Primary Outcome	Secondary End points	Population	Intervention	Duration	Main Findings
Lyon Diet Heart Study	de Lorgeril et al,[6] 1999	France	3 composite outcomes (CO): CO1, cardiovascular death and nonfatal MI; CO2, preceding plus major secondary events (unstable angina, stroke, heart failure, pulmonary or peripheral embolism); CO3, preceding plus minor events requiring hospitalization	—	Men and women with previous MI	Mediterranean-style diet (MD) with high-ALA margarine provided (n = 302) or prudent AHA diet (n = 303)	Mean follow-up 46 mo	MD reduced all events: CO1, RR 0.28 (95% CI: 0.15–0.53); CO2, RR 0.33 (95% CI:0.21–0.52); CO3, RR 0.53 (95% CI: 0.38–0.74)
	de Lorgeril et al,[16] 1994	France	Cardiovascular death and nonfatal MI	Noncardiac deaths and minor events requiring hospitalization	Men and women with previous MI	Mediterranean-style diet (MD) with high-ALA margarine provided (n = 302) or prudent AHA diet (n = 303)	Mean follow-up 27 mo	Cardiac death RR: 0.24 (95% CI: 0.07–0.85) Main end points combined RR: 0.27 (95% CI: 0.12–0.59) Total mortality RR: 0.30 (95% CI: 0.11–0.82)
PREDIMED (Prevención con Dieta Mediterránea)	Estruch et al,[8] 2013	Spain	Composite of cardiovascular death, nonfatal MI, and nonfatal stroke	Stroke, MI, death from cardiovascular causes, and death from any cause	7447 men and women with no cardiovascular disease but T2DM or ≥3 risk factors (smoking, hypertension, elevated LDL-C, low HDL, overweight/obese, or family history of premature CHD)	MD+EVOO (~1 L/wk), MD+nuts (30 g/d: 15 g walnuts, 7.5 g hazelnuts, 7.5 g almonds), or low-fat control diet	Median follow-up 4.8 y	Both MD reduced risk for incidence of major cardiovascular events Unadjusted hazard ratio 0.70 for both MD+EVOO and MD+nuts (95% CI: 0.53 to 0.91 and 0.53 to 0.94, respectively)

Abbreviations: ALA, α-linolenic acid; CHD, coronary heart disease; CI, confidence interval; EVOO, extra-virgin olive oil; MI, myocardial infarction; RR, risk ratio; T2DM, type 2 diabetes mellitus.
Data from Refs.[6,8,16]

Table 4
Studies evaluating the effect of a Mediterranean diet supplemented with nuts or EVOO on cardiovascular risk factors in PREDIMED

Authors,[Ref.] Year	Outcome	Sample Population (N)[a]	Duration	Main Findings
Domenech et al,[52] 2014	24-h ambulatory blood pressure	235	1 y	Both MD+EVOO and MD+nuts reduced 24-h SBP, daytime SBP, and daytime DBP Only MD+EVOO reduced nighttime SBP, 24-h DBP, and nighttime DBP
Salas-Salvado et al,[45] 2014	Incidence of new-onset T2DM	Nondiabetics 3541	4.1 y	Only MD+EVOO reduced diabetes risk
Fito et al,[53] 2014	Heart failure biomarkers	930	1 y	Both MDs reduced plasma N-terminal pro-brain natriuretic peptide Only MD+EVOO reduced oxidized LDL-C and lipoprotein(a)
Sala-Vila et al,[46] 2014	ICA-IMT and plaque height	175	2.4 y	Only MD+nuts resulted in ICA-IMT regression and reduced maximum ICA-IMT and maximum plaque height
Murie-Fernandez et al,[47] 2011	Carotid IMT	187	1 y	Both MDs significantly reduced IMT progression only among participants with baseline IMT ≥ 0.9 mm
Toledo et al,[51] 2013	Blood pressure	Full PREDIMED population 7447	4 y	Both MDs reduced DBP relative to control
Salas-Salvado et al,[44] 2011	Incidence of T2DM	Nondiabetics 418	4 y	52% reduction in diabetes incidence for pooled MD groups
Sola et al,[48] 2011	Apolipoproteins (Apo)	551	3 mo	MD+EVOO reduced ApoB/ApoA-I ratio, reduced ApoB, and increased ApoA-I

Perona et al,[49] 2010	VLDL composition	50	3 mo	Both MDs lowered TG MD+nuts: reduced TC and LDL-C; VLDL-TG species characterized by higher LA MD+EVOO: increased HDL-C, reduced VLDL-C, VLDL-TG content, and TG:apolipoprotein B ratio in VLDL; VLDL-TG species enriched in oleic acid
Mena et al,[50] 2009	Inflammatory biomarkers	106	3 mo	Both MD+EVOO and MD+nuts decreased monocyte expression of CD49d and CD40; decreased interleukin-6 and s-ICAM-1 Only MD+EVOO decreased s-VCAM-1 and CRP
Salas-Salvado et al,[43] 2008	Metabolic Syndrome status	1224	1 y	Only MD+nuts significantly reduced MetSyn prevalence and improved MetSyn reversion
Estruch et al,[42] 2006	Traditional CVD risk factors	772	3 mo	Both MD+EVOO and MD+nuts improved glucose, SBP, TC:HDL, HDL-C, interleukin-6, ICAM-1, and VCAM-1; and improved fasting insulin and HOMA-IR in nondiabetics MD+nuts reduced TC and TG while MD+EVOO reduced DBP and CRP

Abbreviations: DBP, diastolic blood pressure; ICA-IMT, internal carotid artery intima-media thickness; LA, linoleic acid; MD+EVOO, Mediterranean diet supplemented with extra-virgin olive oil; MD+nuts, Mediterranean diet supplemented with nuts; MetSyn, metabolic syndrome; s-ICAM-1, soluble intercellular adhesion molecule 1; s-VCAM, soluble vascular cell adhesion molecule; SBP, systolic blood pressure; T2DM, type 2 diabetes mellitus; TC, total cholesterol; TG, triglycerides.

[a] PREDIMED population consisted of men and women with no cardiovascular disease but type 2 diabetes or ≥3 of the following risk factors: smoking, hypertension, elevated LDL-C, low HDL-C, overweight/obese, or a family history of premature CHD.

Data from Refs.[42–53]

lower total cholesterol/HDL-C ratios compared with the low(er)-fat group (−0.38 and −0.26, respectively). In addition, the Mediterranean diet with nuts reduced fasting glucose (−5.4 mg/dL), SBP (−7.1 mm Hg), DBP (−2.6 mm Hg), and TG concentrations (−13 mg/dL) relative to the low(er)-fat diet.[42] The Mediterranean diet with olive oil also reduced fasting glucose (−7.0 mg/dL), SBP (−5.9 mm Hg), and DBP (−1.6 mm Hg), but did not reduce triglyceride concentrations compared with the low(er)-fat diet. The trial was stopped early because of the significant clinical benefits observed for the combined CVD outcomes end point of stroke, MI, or death from cardiovascular outcomes.[8] Participants in both the higher nut and higher EVOO diets experienced an approximate 30% reduction in the primary end point relative to the low(er) fat diet group.[8] When the individual components of the combined CVD outcome were analyzed separately, only the reduction in stroke risk reached significance (Mediterranean diet + EVOO: hazard ratio 0.67, 95% confidence interval [CI] 0.46–0.98; hazard ratio for Mediterranean diet + nuts: 0.54, 95% CI 0.35–0.84). It also is important to note that the macronutrient composition of the 3 diet treatments were somewhat similar, with only a 4 percentage point difference in total fat intake between the low(er)fat and Mediterranean diet groups. The Lyon Diet Heart Study and PREDIMED remain the only long-term intervention studies of a Mediterranean-style dietary pattern, and demonstrate significant improvements in cardiovascular mortality (**Table 3**).

Additional analyses of PREDIMED subcohorts have further demonstrated the benefits of Mediterranean-style diets containing nuts and/or EVOO on various CVD risk factors (**Table 4**). After 1 year of follow-up, only the Mediterranean diet group supplemented with nuts reduced the prevalence of metabolic syndrome.[43] After 4 years of follow-up, both Mediterranean diets reduced the incidence of diabetes by 52% compared with a low(er)-fat diet in individuals with high CVD risk.[44] However, in a subsequent analysis of a larger nondiabetic population, only the Mediterranean diet supplemented with EVOO reduced the risk of new-onset type 2 diabetes.[45] Additional follow-up studies reported reductions in carotid intima-media thickness,[46,47] apolipoproteins,[48] very low-density lipoprotein (VLDL) cholesterol,[49] inflammatory biomarkers,[50] and improvements in DBP,[51] ambulatory blood pressure,[52] and heart failure biomarkers.[53] It is interesting that supplementation with nuts versus EVOO elicited beneficial effects on different CVD risk factors, without a clear trend indicating whether one dietary pattern was more effective. This finding may reflect differences in the bioactives provided by nuts and EVOO.

SUMMARY

Results from these clinical trials, particularly PREDIMED, provide convincing evidence that a Mediterranean-style dietary pattern is effective for improving both cardiovascular outcomes and multiple CVD risk factors. Dietary patterns such as the Mediterranean diet result in multiple changes in nutrient consumption that most likely act in an additive, or even synergistic, manner. If these healthy dietary patterns can be sustained over the long term, the evidence base indicates that CVD risk can be markedly reduced. Even small dietary modifications can have a clinically significant benefit. The primary and secondary analyses of PREDIMED demonstrate that both EVOO and mixed nuts can be effectively incorporated into a Mediterranean-style diet to provide substantial cardiovascular benefits.

The addition of the Mediterranean diet to the list of evidence-based dietary patterns may help individuals achieve better long-term adherence to a cardioprotective diet if the composition of the Mediterranean diet more closely aligns with their cultural and personal preferences than other recommended dietary patterns. Significant dietary changes can be achieved in the short term, but dietary and lifestyle modifications can be difficult to sustain. Consequently, waning compliance results in diminished CVD risk reduction. Thus, a nutrient-dense dietary pattern that provides options to reflect personal preferences may help patients maintain a healthy diet and achieve maximal reduction in CVD risk.

A Mediterranean-style dietary pattern reflects most food and nutrient goals recommended by the DGA 2010 and 2013 AHA/ACC Lifestyle Guideline. Minor modifications to the traditional Mediterranean dietary pattern can be made to reduce sodium and saturated fat intake and meet current dietary recommendations. Emphasizing low-fat or fat-free dairy in place of full-fat cheeses, removing skin from poultry, and emphasizing nuts high in unsaturated fat (eg, walnuts, almonds, hazelnuts, and pistachios) would further reduce saturated fat intake and promote LDL-C reduction, a primary goal of the AHA/ACC Lifestyle Guideline. Although it is not the primary dietary pattern recommended, implementation of a Mediterranean-style diet improves cardiovascular outcomes even in the absence of reductions in traditional CVD risk factors. In addition to cardiovascular outcomes, numerous other studies have demonstrated reductions in multiple, major CVD risk factors, including lipids and lipoproteins, blood pressure, and body weight, which would be expected to further decrease CVD risk. Thus, it is possible that future dietary guidelines will place greater emphasis on the Mediterranean diet as a dietary pattern for the prevention and treatment of CVD, in addition to other chronic diseases.

REFERENCES

1. Page IH, Stare FJ, Corcoran AC, et al. Atherosclerosis and the fat content of the diet. J Am Med Assoc 1957;164(18):2048–51.
2. US Department of Agriculture, US Department of Health and Human Services. Dietary guidelines for Americans 2010. 7th edition. Washington, DC: US Government Printing Office; 2010.
3. Eckel RH, Jakicic JM, Ard JD, et al. 2013 AHA/ACC guideline on lifestyle management to reduce cardiovascular risk: a report of the American College of Cardiology/American Heart Association Task Force on practice guidelines. J Am Coll Cardiol 2014;63(25 Pt B):2960–84.
4. Appel LJ, Moore TJ, Obarzanek E, et al. A clinical trial of the effects of dietary patterns on blood pressure. N Engl J Med 1997;336(16):1117–24.
5. Sacks FM, Svetkey LP, Vollmer WM, et al, DASH-Sodium Collaborative Research Group. Effects on blood pressure of reduced dietary sodium and the Dietary Approaches to Stop Hypertension (DASH) diet. N Engl J Med 2001;344(1):3–10.
6. de Lorgeril M, Salen P, Martin JL, et al. Mediterranean diet, traditional risk factors, and the rate of cardiovascular complications after myocardial infarction: final report of the Lyon Diet Heart Study. Circulation 1999;99(6):779–85.
7. Vincent-Baudry S, Defoort C, Gerber M, et al. The Medi-RIVAGE study: reduction of cardiovascular disease risk factors after a 3-mo intervention with a Mediterranean-type diet or a low-fat diet. Am J Clin Nutr 2005;82(5):964–71.
8. Estruch R, Ros E, Salas-Salvado J, et al. Primary prevention of cardiovascular disease with a Mediterranean diet. N Engl J Med 2013;368(14):1279–90.
9. Appel LJ, Sacks FM, Carey VJ, et al. Effects of protein, monounsaturated fat, and carbohydrate intake on blood pressure and serum lipids: results of the OmniHeart randomized trial. JAMA 2005;294(19):2455–64.
10. Mozaffarian D, Appel LJ, Van Horn L. Components of a cardioprotective diet: new insights. Circulation 2011;123(24):2870–91.

11. Lichtenstein AH, Appel LJ, Brands M, et al. Diet and lifestyle recommendations revision 2006: a scientific statement from the American Heart Association Nutrition Committee. Circulation 2006;114(1):82–96.

12. Van Horn L, McCoin M, Kris-Etherton PM, et al. The evidence for dietary prevention and treatment of cardiovascular disease. J Am Diet Assoc 2008;108(2): 287–331.

13. Bach-Faig A, Berry EM, Lairon D, et al. Mediterranean diet pyramid today. Science and cultural updates. Public Health Nutr 2011;14(12A):2274–84.

14. Keys A. Coronary heart disease in seven countries. Circulation 1970;41:I1–211.

15. Keys A, Menotti A, Karvonen MJ, et al. The diet and 15-year death rate in the seven countries study. Am J Epidemiol 1986;124(6):903–15.

16. de Lorgeril M, Renaud S, Mamelle N, et al. Mediterranean alpha-linolenic acid-rich diet in secondary prevention of coronary heart disease. Lancet 1994;343(8911): 1454–9.

17. Sofi F, Cesari F, Abbate R, et al. Adherence to Mediterranean diet and health status: meta-analysis. BMJ 2008;337:a1344.

18. Sofi F, Abbate R, Gensini GF, et al. Accruing evidence on benefits of adherence to the Mediterranean diet on health: an updated systematic review and meta-analysis. Am J Clin Nutr 2010;92(5):1189–96.

19. Sofi F, Macchi C, Abbate R, et al. Mediterranean diet and health status: an updated meta-analysis and a proposal for a literature-based adherence score. Public Health Nutr 2013;1–14.

20. Mente A, de Koning L, Shannon HS, et al. A systematic review of the evidence supporting a causal link between dietary factors and coronary heart disease. Arch Intern Med 2009;169(7):659–69.

21. Chiuve SE, Fung TT, Rexrode KM, et al. Adherence to a low-risk, healthy lifestyle and risk of sudden cardiac death among women. JAMA 2011;306(1):62–9.

22. Kastorini CM, Milionis HJ, Esposito K, et al. The effect of Mediterranean diet on metabolic syndrome and its components: a meta-analysis of 50 studies and 534,906 individuals. J Am Coll Cardiol 2011;57(11):1299–313.

23. Grosso G, Mistretta A, Frigiola A, et al. Mediterranean diet and cardiovascular risk factors: a systematic review. Crit Rev Food Sci Nutr 2014;54(5):593–610.

24. Martinez-Gonzalez MA, Bes-Rastrollo M. Dietary patterns, Mediterranean diet, and cardiovascular disease. Curr Opin Lipidol 2014;25(1):20–6.

25. Nordmann AJ, Suter-Zimmermann K, Bucher HC, et al. Meta-analysis comparing Mediterranean to low-fat diets for modification of cardiovascular risk factors. Am J Med 2011;124(9):841–51.e2.

26. Serra-Majem L, Roman B, Estruch R. Scientific evidence of interventions using the Mediterranean diet: a systematic review. Nutr Rev 2006;64(2 Pt 2):S27–47.

27. Elhayany A, Lustman A, Abel R, et al. A low carbohydrate Mediterranean diet improves cardiovascular risk factors and diabetes control among overweight patients with type 2 diabetes mellitus: a 1-year prospective randomized intervention study. Diabetes Obes Metab 2010;12(3):204–9.

28. Bravo-Herrera MD, Lopez-Miranda J, Marin C, et al. Tissue factor expression is decreased in monocytes obtained from blood during Mediterranean or high carbohydrate diets. Nutr Metab Cardiovasc Dis 2004;14(3):128–32.

29. Esposito K, Marfella R, Ciotola M, et al. Effect of a Mediterranean-style diet on endothelial dysfunction and markers of vascular inflammation in the metabolic syndrome: a randomized trial. JAMA 2004;292(12):1440–6.

30. Ferro-Luzzi A, Strazzullo P, Scaccini C, et al. Changing the Mediterranean diet: effects on blood lipids. Am J Clin Nutr 1984;40(5):1027–37.

31. Rodriguez-Villar C, Perez-Heras A, Mercade I, et al. Comparison of a high-carbohydrate and a high-monounsaturated fat, olive oil-rich diet on the susceptibility of LDL to oxidative modification in subjects with Type 2 diabetes mellitus. Diabet Med 2004;21(2):142–9.
32. Esposito K, Maiorino MI, Ciotola M, et al. Effects of a Mediterranean-style diet on the need for antihyperglycemic drug therapy in patients with newly diagnosed type 2 diabetes: a randomized trial. Ann Intern Med 2009; 151(5):306–14.
33. Toobert DJ, Glasgow RE, Strycker LA, et al. Biologic and quality-of-life outcomes from the Mediterranean Lifestyle Program: a randomized clinical trial. Diabetes Care 2003;26(8):2288–93.
34. Stachowska E, Wesolowska T, Olszewska M, et al. Elements of Mediterranean diet improve oxidative status in blood of kidney graft recipients. Br J Nutr 2005;93(3):345–52.
35. Sondergaard E, Moller JE, Egstrup K. Effect of dietary intervention and lipid-lowering treatment on brachial vasoreactivity in patients with ischemic heart disease and hypercholesterolemia. Am Heart J 2003;145(5):E19.
36. Singh N, Graves J, Taylor PD, et al. Effects of a 'healthy' diet and of acute and long-term vitamin C on vascular function in healthy older subjects. Cardiovasc Res 2002;56(1):118–25.
37. Fuentes F, Lopez-Miranda J, Sanchez E, et al. Mediterranean and low-fat diets improve endothelial function in hypercholesterolemic men. Ann Intern Med 2001;134(12):1115–9.
38. Strazzullo P, Ferro-Luzzi A, Siani A, et al. Changing the Mediterranean diet: effects on blood pressure. J Hypertens 1986;4(4):407–12.
39. Tuttle KR, Shuler LA, Packard DP, et al. Comparison of low-fat versus Mediterranean-style dietary intervention after first myocardial infarction (from The Heart Institute of Spokane Diet Intervention and Evaluation Trial). Am J Cardiol 2008;101(11):1523–30.
40. Michalsen A, Lehmann N, Pithan C, et al. Mediterranean diet has no effect on markers of inflammation and metabolic risk factors in patients with coronary artery disease. Eur J Clin Nutr 2006;60(4):478–85.
41. Perez-Jimenez F, Lopez-Miranda J, Pinillos MD, et al. A Mediterranean and a high-carbohydrate diet improve glucose metabolism in healthy young persons. Diabetologia 2001;44(11):2038–43.
42. Estruch R, Martinez-Gonzalez MA, Corella D, et al. Effects of a Mediterranean-style diet on cardiovascular risk factors: a randomized trial. Ann Intern Med 2006;145(1):1–11.
43. Salas-Salvado J, Fernandez-Ballart J, Ros E, et al. Effect of a Mediterranean diet supplemented with nuts on metabolic syndrome status: one-year results of the PREDIMED randomized trial. Arch Intern Med 2008;168(22):2449–58.
44. Salas-Salvadó J, Bulló M, Babio N, et al. Reduction in the incidence of type 2 diabetes with the Mediterranean diet: results of the PREDIMED-Reus nutrition intervention randomized trial. Diabetes Care 2011;34(1):14.
45. Salas-Salvado J, Bullo M, Estruch R, et al. Prevention of diabetes with Mediterranean diets: a subgroup analysis of a randomized trial. Ann Intern Med 2014; 160(1):1–10.
46. Sala-Vila A, Romero-Mamani ES, Gilabert R, et al. Changes in ultrasound-assessed carotid intima-media thickness and plaque with a Mediterranean diet: a substudy of the PREDIMED trial. Arterioscler Thromb Vasc Biol 2014; 34(2):439–45.

47. Murie-Fernandez M, Irimia P, Toledo E, et al. Carotid intima-media thickness changes with Mediterranean diet: a randomized trial (PREDIMED-Navarra). Atherosclerosis 2011;219(1):158–62.

48. Sola R, Fito M, Estruch R, et al. Effect of a traditional Mediterranean diet on apolipoproteins B, A-I, and their ratio: a randomized, controlled trial. Atherosclerosis 2011;218(1):174–80.

49. Perona JS, Covas MI, Fito M, et al. Reduction in systemic and VLDL triacylglycerol concentration after a 3-month Mediterranean-style diet in high-cardiovascular-risk subjects. J Nutr Biochem 2010;21(9):892–8.

50. Mena MP, Sacanella E, Vazquez-Agell M, et al. Inhibition of circulating immune cell activation: a molecular antiinflammatory effect of the Mediterranean diet. Am J Clin Nutr 2009;89(1):248–56.

51. Toledo E, Hu FB, Estruch R, et al. Effect of the Mediterranean diet on blood pressure in the PREDIMED trial: results from a randomized controlled trial. BMC Med 2013;11:207.

52. Domenech M, Roman P, Lapetra J, et al. Mediterranean diet reduces 24-hour ambulatory blood pressure, blood glucose, and lipids: one-year randomized, clinical trial. Hypertension 2014;64(1):69–76.

53. Fito M, Estruch R, Salas-Salvado J, et al. Effect of the Mediterranean diet on heart failure biomarkers: a randomized sample from the PREDIMED trial. Eur J Heart Fail 2014;16(5):543–50.

54. Ros E, Nunez I, Perez-Heras A, et al. A walnut diet improves endothelial function in hypercholesterolemic subjects: a randomized crossover trial. Circulation 2004;109(13):1609–14.

55. Mezzano D, Leighton F, Martinez C, et al. Complementary effects of Mediterranean diet and moderate red wine intake on haemostatic cardiovascular risk factors. Eur J Clin Nutr 2001;55(6):444–51.

56. Zambon D, Sabate J, Munoz S, et al. Substituting walnuts for monounsaturated fat improves the serum lipid profile of hypercholesterolemic men and women. A randomized crossover trial. Ann Intern Med 2000;132(7):538–46.

Pediatric Lipid Management

An Earlier Approach

Justin P. Zachariah, MD, MPH[a,b,*], Philip K. Johnson, BS[a,b]

KEYWORDS

- Pediatrics • Lipids • Atherosclerosis • Dyslipidemia

KEY POINTS

- Numerous long-term observational cohort studies show that subclinical atherosclerosis is a progressive disease that arises in childhood and continues through the adulthood.
- Deficiencies in targeted lipid screening to identify high-risk individuals led the 2011 National Heart, Lung and Blood Institute Expert Panel for Pediatric Cardiovascular Disease (CVD) Risk Reduction to recommend universal screening.
- Amid concerns that extended screening may induce inappropriate treatment, pharmacotherapy is restricted to patients with genetic dyslipidemias and multiple high-risk CVD factors.
- This article summarizes the current guidelines, enumerates challenges to the guidelines, and suggests future directions.

INTRODUCTION

Although adult cardiovascular disease (CVD) mortality has been curtailed primarily from improvements in atherosclerotic risk factor treatment, an alarming countervailing trend dominates the present and future of CVD: obesity, obesity-related dyslipidemia, and type 2 diabetes.[1–6] Children offer a prime opportunity to continue CVD risk factor reduction and address emerging trends, especially dyslipidemia.

There are 4 general classes of pediatric dyslipidemias:

- Medication-related dyslipidemia
- Dyslipidemia related to lifestyle factors

Disclosures: The authors have no financial conflicts of interest. This work was supported by NHLBI Career Development Award K23 HL111335 (J.P. Zachariah). No funding sources had any role in the design, writing, editing, or decision to publish any part of this work.
[a] Department of Cardiology, Boston Children's Hospital, 300 Longwood Avenue, Boston, MA 02115, USA; [b] Department of Pediatrics, Harvard Medical School, 300 Longwood Avenue, Boston, MA 02115, USA
* Corresponding author. Department of Cardiology, Boston Children's Hospital, 300 Longwood Avenue, Boston, MA 02115.
E-mail address: justin.zachariah@childrens.harvard.edu

Endocrinol Metab Clin N Am 43 (2014) 981–992
http://dx.doi.org/10.1016/j.ecl.2014.08.004
0889-8529/14/$ – see front matter © 2014 Elsevier Inc. All rights reserved.

- Genetic dyslipidemia
- Dyslipidemia secondary to a medical condition.

There are 3 chief genetic dyslipidemias (**Table 1**).

- Familial hypercholesterolemia (FH). FH is an autosomal dominant disorder that interferes with either apolipoprotein B (ApoB) assembly or the receptor-mediated clearance of low-density lipoprotein cholesterol (LDL-C) in roughly 1 in 500 persons with heterozygosity or 1 in a million homozygotes.[7–10] However, homozygotes frequently develop xanthelasmas of the canthi, xanthomas on the extensor surfaces of limb joints, arcus senilis of the eye, and internal consequences, including myocardial infarction and ischemic cardiomyopathy, often in the first 2 decades of life. The heterozygous phenotype predisposes to early atherosclerosis and is more common than, and as treatable as, any disorder within national newborn screening programs.
- Familial combined hyperlipidemia. Familial combined hyperlipidemia is another genetic dyslipidemia with high LDL-C and triglycerides (TGs), but lacks the degree of TG increase necessary to trigger pancreatitis. It confers CVD risks nearly as high as FH and may be as prevalent as 1% of the population.[11,12]
- Familial severe hypertriglyceridemia (HTG). Although 1 in 600 individuals have severe HTG (defined as TG>10 mmol/L or 885 mg/dL),[13] much of this is caused by environment and lifestyle. Genetic or familial HTG has many implicated genes, but the most common is homozygous autosomal recessive loss of function mutations in lipoprotein lipase or apolipoprotein C2 and occurs in 1 in 1 × 10⁵ individuals.[13,14] Hindered degradation of TG leads to significantly increased serum TG.[15,16] At levels of more than 1000 mg/dL, the risk of acutely life-threatening pancreatitis increases. However, risk stratification by TG level is inadequate because many lipid providers follow persons with TG greater than 2000 mg/dL who have never had pancreatitis. Despite this uncertainty, prompt treatment is recommended.[17]

Suggested responses to pediatric dyslipidemias include, but are not limited to, removing a causative agent, lifestyle modification, treating an underlying medical condition, and in severe cases pharmacotherapy. Each of these therapeutic maneuvers is intended to accomplish 2 important goals: preventing acute pancreatitis in individuals with very increased TGs levels and preventing atherosclerotic CVD later in life.

Table 1 Prominent genetic dyslipidemias in children			
Dyslipidemia	**Abnormal Lipid Fraction**	**Prevalence Estimate**	**Predominant Mechanism**
Familial hypercholesterolemia	High LDL-C	Heterozygotes, 1 in 500 Homozygotes, 1 in million	Decreased LDL-C clearance
Familial combined hypercholesterolemia	High LDL-C and high triglycerides/ VLDL	1 in 100[11]	Increased ApoB production
Familial severe hypertriglyceridemia	High triglycerides/ VLDL	1 in 100,000[13]	Decreased triglyceride/ VLDL degradation

Abbreviations: ApoB, apolipoprotein B; LDL-C, low-density lipoprotein cholesterol; VLDL, very low-density lipoprotein.

Childhood is also a key period for progress because children are susceptible to deleterious lifestyle influences; are directly affected by CVD risk factors; already accumulate atherosclerotic phenotypic changes; are more malleable to lifestyle habit alterations to avoid CVD risk factors; and, through internal motivation and/or support form guardians or peers, have the capacity to treat CVD risk factors through lifestyle modification alone. The clinical encounter offers an opportunity to leverage abnormal laboratory results into a multifaceted cardiometabolic remedy. In a recent study of medical providers caring for children, 74% thought that lipid screening and treatment would reduce future CVD outcomes. Despite this belief, only 16% universally screened their patients, 54% selectively screened, and 34% did not screen at all.[18] These data underscore the need to engage providers.

The National Heart, Lung and Blood Institute (NHLBI) Expert Panel on Integrated Guidelines for Cardiovascular Disease Health and Risk Reduction in Children and Adolescents released their guidelines in November 2011, unifying previously disjointed aspects of CVD prevention, including physical activity, nutrition, obesity, blood pressure, lipids, and tobacco use, under a singular aegis and updated these domains with a comprehensive review of relevant data.[19] In compiling these revised recommendations, the NHLBI guidelines lengthen the reach of CVD prevention to an earlier, more plastic stage of life.

THE GUIDELINES: FRAMEWORK AND SYNOPSIS

CVD risk factor modification can be subdivided into primary, secondary, and primordial prevention.[20] Primary prevention is the treatment of risk factors to avoid the first event, secondary prevention is the evasion of recurrent cardiovascular events in patients with a history of CVD, and primordial prevention is intervention to prevent CVD risk factors from arising at all.[21] In order to inhibit the development of CVD risk factors, the NHLBI Integrated Guidelines make precise, developmentally appropriate suggestions interweaving CVD risk factor prevention within general pediatric practice. The screening and treatment sections focus on the premise that CVD risk factors must be centered on the child's aggregate combination of cardiac risks, rather than any particular risk factor.

It is well recognized that atherosclerotic abnormalities arise in childhood, that these changes are related to the presence of CVD risk factors, and that risk factors in adults are directly related to cardiac events in a continuous fashion.[22–26] However, when the population is "sick", as Geoffrey Rose[27] described, what is to be done? Nationally representative pediatric data show that overweight and obesity increase the relative risk of increased LDL cholesterol (LDL-C); however, approximately 45% of all adolescents with high LDL-C are of normal weight, suggesting that CVD risk factors are widespread. It is therefore essential that the proposed suggestions be scaled to the population level because fixating on excess weight misses almost half the problem.[28]

It is also clear that population-wide interventions can be successful, as shown by tobacco use reduction. Tobacco use reduction has been achieved through mobilizing public sentiment; initiating economic disincentives; and placing restrictions on the procurement, advertisement, and use of tobacco products. Similar efforts to reduce the causes of hyperlipidemia, hypertension, or obesity meet entrenched resistance from the lack of data supporting secondhand harm from lifestyle behaviors and trepidation about the freedom of personal choice. Protecting children from circumstances that ultimately lead to CVD risk factors may be more readily accepted because their lifestyle choices are appropriately constrained by caregivers since they are less proficient in making their own healthy choices. Therefore the guidelines make primordial prevention recommendations for all children and primary prevention recommendations for affected children, including those with dyslipidemia.

Primordial Prevention Recommendations

1. The Integrated Guidelines seek to perform population-level prevention through each child. Nutrition recommendations include:
   - Breastfeeding for the first 12 months
   - Restricting calories derived from milk fat and fruit juice
   - After age 2 years, adherence to the Cardiovascular Health Integrated Lifestyle Diet (CHILD-1) diet[19]
2. Tobacco abolition is recommended from infancy through childhood and adolescence
3. Universal recommendations with respect to activity and inactivity consist of:
   - Consistent active play in toddlerhood
   - One hour per day of moderate to vigorous exercise in older children and adolescents
   - Inactive screen time is fully discouraged before age 2 years
   - Screen time is restricted to less than 2 hours per day in older children

The guidelines advance, endorse, and stress this population-level approach to CVD risk factor mitigation as the new norm for US children. It is thought that this combination of interventions will simultaneously protect against incident dyslipidemia, diabetes, hypertension, and obesity.

Primary Prevention Recommendations

The Integrated Guidelines refine, extend, and combine previous guidelines from the American Academy of Pediatrics (AAP) 2008 guidelines on dyslipidemia detection.[29,30] These prior efforts advocated for screening for lipid disorders in patients with high-risk medical conditions and/or abnormal family histories and pharmacologic management of severe pediatric lipid disorders. The 2011 NHLBI guidelines expand the AAP cholesterol guidelines by recommending universal screening to enhance the detection of young patients with FH who are subject to atherosclerotic events in early adulthood.

1. Universal screening can be initiated with either:
   a. A calculated nonfasting non–high-density lipoprotein cholesterol (HDL-C) level, and HDL-C level, or
   b. A fasting lipid panel
2. Abnormal levels should be confirmed with a repeated fasting test, especially for TG irregularities
3. Targeted lipid screening can occur
   a. At any time after age 2 years for children at high atherosclerotic risk (**Box 1**)[19]
   b. At the provider's preference, or
   c. At the family's discretion
4. Very high levels of TG or LDL-C ($\geq$500 mg/dL and $\geq$250 mg/dL, respectively) trigger a referral to a lipid specialist in order to manage genetic dyslipidemias

The NHLBI guidelines are designed to set thresholds to reflect the well-documented age-specific distribution of lipid levels in the hope of increasing the number of children eligible for attention but constraining the number eligible for medication. They also mirror the 3 category groupings of the Adult Treatment Panel III/National Cholesterol Education Program in defining acceptable lipid values (**Table 2**).

Box 1
Risk factor definitions for dyslipidemia algorithms

Family history

In parent, grandparent, aunt, or uncle a history of myocardial infarction, angina, coronary artery bypass graft/stent/angioplasty, or sudden cardiac death before age 55 years in men or 65 years in women

High-level risk factors

Hypertension requiring therapy

Current cigarette smoker

Body mass index (BMI) greater than 97%

High-risk conditions

   Diabetes mellitus, type 1 or 2

   After heart transplant

   Chronic kidney disease

   End-stage renal disease

   After renal transplant

   Kawasaki disease with coronary aneurysms

Moderate-level risk factors

Hypertension not requiring medication

BMI greater than 95% but less than or equal to 97%

HDL-C less than 40 mg/dL

Moderate-risk condition

   Chronic inflammatory disease

   Human immunodeficiency virus infection

   Nephrotic syndrome

   Kawasaki disease without coronary aneurysm

Data from Expert panel on integrated guidelines for cardiovascular health and risk reduction in children and adolescents: summary report. Pediatrics 2011;128(Suppl 5):S237.

Treatment of CVD risk factors is an essential part of the NHLBI guidelines. It is also clear that CVD risk factors are modifiable. Adult cohort studies show that 90% of coronary heart disease (CHD) and incident stroke and were attributable to modifiable risk factors.[31–34] Temporal trends show that smoking rates have decreased in adults, and, in American children, cholesterol levels seem to be declining as well.[35,36] According to recent randomized controlled trials in adults with type 2 diabetes, coronary disease with systolic heart failure, and chronic stable angina, aggressive CVD risk factor modification was as effective as invasive revascularization in averting CVD events.[37–39] In contrast, 30-year global trends show that obesity prevalence is increasing and cholesterol levels are worsening.[40,41] Therefore, clinicians can be confident that CVD risk factors are modifiable in both the positive and negative directions. Therapy in children is justified by direct links between risk factors in adolescence and atherosclerotic disorders, CVD risk factor stability from childhood to adulthood, and the ability of pediatric risk factors to predict adverse vascular changes and CVD events, even after adult CVD risk factor level adjustment.[24,25,42–46]

Table 2 Lipid parameter classification			
Category	Acceptable	Borderline	High
Total cholesterol	<170	170–199	≥200
LDL-C	<110	110–129	≥130
TG			
0–9 y	<75	75–99	≥100
10–19 y	<90	90–129	≥130
Non–HDL-C	<120	120–144	≥145
ApoB	<90	90–109	≥110
Category	Acceptable	Borderline	Low
HDL-C	>45	40–45	<40
ApoA-I	>120	115–120	<115

Abbreviation: ApoA-I, apolipoprotein A-I.
Data from Expert panel on integrated guidelines for cardiovascular health and risk reduction in children and adolescents: summary report. Pediatrics 2011;128(Suppl 5):S240.

The Expert Panel recommends that children with lipid disorders partake of dyslipidemia-determined special diets for at least 6 months and diminish obesity if appropriate. After 6 months of lifestyle modification, triggers referral to lipid specialists to consider statin initiation. The presence of multiple risks or higher intensity risks progressively decreases the LDL-C threshold to initiate statin pharmacotherapy, and decreases the goal LDL-C concentration on treatment.[47–51] The key components of TG treatment center on simple carbohydrate intake reduction, increased omega-3 intake through fish consumption or omega-3 supplements, or severe reduction in fat intake as appropriate. If these maneuvers are ineffective in reducing TG levels sufficiently to mitigate the risk of pancreatitis, referral to a lipid specialist for non-HDL reduction through lipid pharmacotherapy is advised.

CHALLENGES TO THE LIPID MANAGEMENT GUIDELINES
Universal Screening

The most controversial topic raised by the integrated panel has been a call for universal lipid screening, which is intended to improve identification of genetic dyslipidemias like heterozygous FH. FH seems to fulfill 1968 World Health Organization criteria: it occurs in 1 in 500 births, silently leads to highly increased LDL-C over a person's life, manifests as CVD mortality events in young adulthood, and the combination of lipid-lowering drugs and lifestyle modification seems to attenuate the excess risk.[52] Approximately 20% of girls and 50% of boys with FH heterozygosity will have a coronary event before age 50 years.[7,8,53] Although previous guidelines restricted screening to only those children with an increased risk of dyslipidemia based on personal health features or family history, studies show that reliance on family history of CVD events or high lipid levels may miss 30% to 60% of afflicted children because of a lack of knowledge about family history, lack of understanding about lipid levels, the ability of medications presently available to profoundly reduce or prevent CVD events in affected adults, or a parent's refusal to be tested for cholesterol level.[9,54–57] Focusing on children treats them as individuals worthy of care independent of the dependability of their parents and, in a reverse cascade, may boost identification of family members with FH who might not have been detected otherwise.

The disadvantages of universal screening should not be glossed over.[58–60] Children could be incorrectly labeled as abnormal from a nonfasting lipid screening, because CVD risk factors fluctuate throughout childhood and adulthood. However, also similar to adults, isolated lipid measurements in childhood predict atherosclerosis in adulthood.[24,25,42] The guidelines recommend using high thresholds to designate abnormal levels in conjunction with taking the average of multiple lipid values to help avoid misclassification and errors from regression to the mean. It is highly likely that a small number will be inappropriately labeled as FH despite following the guidelines in obtaining 2 more fasting lipid panels. More data must be gathered to assess the negative and positive biological, social, and psychological effects of this screening approach.

Lifestyle Dyslipidemias

The panel acknowledges the probability of discovering lifestyle-driven dyslipidemias and advocates that such children should receive medical attention. Critics note that lipid values fluctuate during childhood and that obesity increases an individual's risk for having abnormal lipid values. With this information they object to classifying a multitude of children, who are already psychologically vulnerable from an abnormal weight label, with an abnormal cholesterol label. If the goal is to lose weight, failure is common and makes the child feel even worse.[58–60]

Although obesity increases the risk of accruing lifestyle-induced dyslipidemias, note that a large proportion of dyslipidemic children are of normal weight, and the most patients who are of abnormal weight are not dyslipidemic.[28] In a related analysis that may parallel efforts in lipid management, detecting and treating abnormal weight with the goal of modifying blood pressure–related CVD did not seem to be a cost-effective way to prevent CVD outcomes.[61] Although the origins of both derive from suboptimal diets and activity levels, dyslipidemia and excess weight are not synonymous. Specific lifestyle modification can modify dyslipidemia without affecting weight immediately.[62–65] As described in the guidelines, for example, the avoidance of simple carbohydrates is not expected to significantly alter LDL-C, but may be useful in hindering insulin resistance mediated by high TG. These dyslipidemia-specific dietary instructions are effective but onerous for families and so should not be applied to the entire population. On the contrary, recent adult meta-analytical data on the effects of dietary saturated fat on CVD and CHD risk outcomes in prospective adult cohort studies suggested that dietary saturated fat was not associated with increased CVD or CHD risk.[11] However, a broad-based adult cohort is not equivalent to a population presenting early in life with markedly abnormal lipid values, and thus the data cannot be generalized to pediatric dyslipidemia. In addition, the CHILD-1 diet recommended for all children without dyslipidemias safely encourages moderation in simple carbohydrates, processed foods, and saturated fat, as well as encouraging consumption of vegetables and lean proteins, which is widely accepted as a sensible approach.[19] In addition, when motivated to avoid medication, youth and families may become more engaged.

By extension, critics are concerned about lifestyle dyslipidemic patients being loosely prescribed statins. The NHLBI panel instead mandates lifestyle alterations as the primary response. Only after this has been assiduously exhausted and additional CVD risks are also present can pharmacotherapy be considered, preferably under a lipid specialist's guidance. This advice is distinctly at odds with treatment patterns among adult providers. The most recent evidence on lipid-lowering therapy indicates that the number of children being treated is grossly inadequate.[66,67] Contrary to popular fears, the guidelines advocate against the indiscriminate distribution of statin drugs to obese children.

Lipid-lowering Treatment

The main criticisms of pediatric lipid pharmacotherapy in general are:

- Invocation of 10-year CVD risk calculators to show that children are inherently low risk
- Lack of data on the benefits of childhood treatment
- Lack of long-term safety data

It is important to recall that the primary intended pediatric recipients of lipid-lowering medications are those with FH. It is improper to use the Framingham 10-year risk calculator on those with genetic dyslipidemia. The Framingham calculator is intended for and derived from a general population cohort, not a high-risk diagnosis such as FH. For example, inputting a cholesterol value of more than 320 mg/dL into the online calculator results in an error message requesting a smaller value. A more suitable risk assessment is family history data in patients with FH showing 50% and 20% risk of coronary events in men and women less than 50 years of age, respectively.[7,8,68]

The criticism regarding lack of long-term data is well taken. The guidelines outline existing data regarding the efficacy and tolerability of statins in reducing LDL-C. However, there are neither studies on the ability of statin therapy started in youth to reduce CVD events nor long-term safety studies, because the logistical complexity and cost of clinical trials following large numbers of patients over several decades are impractical. A recent meta-analysis of placebo adult randomized controlled trials compared the effect of short-term lipid-lowering agents versus naturally occurring LDL-C–lowering genetic mutations on CVD events.[51] This elegant study revealed that CVD prevention per unit LDL-C decrease was several times more effective by genetic polymorphism than by pharmacologic intervention, implying that the amount of time spent at a reduced LDL-C concentration was the leading feature of additional CVD protection. Furthermore, sequence variations in the *PCSK9* gene, which is known to reduce LDL-C, caused 88% and 47% reductions in cardiac disease in African American and white populations.[18] These findings are also in accord with anthropologic epidemiology, which shows lower rates of CVD in cultures with habitually low LDL-C on a population basis.[69,70]

Critics of the guidelines cite unforeseen side effects from other medicines in the past as a reason to avoid a hypothetical pediatric-specific adverse event for lipid-lowering medicine. In contrast, the volume of patient data from statin therapy in adults and children is overwhelming and argues against additional adverse events beyond the well-described myotoxicity, emerging risks regarding incident diabetes mellitus, and possible risk of hepatoxicity.[47–49,71] When family history involves early and severe CVD in a parent, the discussion about treatment takes on a greater sense of urgency. Although the described risks are important to consider, the preponderance of data support the use of lipid-lowering medication in children affected by FH. However, the decision to treat an affected child is always a collaborative one between provider, parent, and child.

SUMMARY

The NHLBI Expert Panel Integrated Guidelines promote the prevention of CVD events by encouraging healthy behaviors in all children, screening and treatment of children with genetic dyslipidemias, usage of specific lifestyle modifications, and limited administration of lipid pharmacotherapy in children with the highest CVD risk. These recommendations place children in the center of the fight against future CVD.

Pediatric providers may be in a position to shift the focus of CVD prevention from trimming multiple risk factors to attacking the roots of CVD.

ADDITIONAL RESOURCES

Centers for Disease Control resources on obesity. Available at:http://www.cdc.gov/obesity/resources/index.html.

2011 NHLBI integrated guidelines for cardiovascular health and risk reduction in children and adolescents. Available at: http://www.nhlbi.nih.gov/health-pro/guidelines/current/cardiovascular-health-pediatric-guidelines/index.htm.

REFERENCES

1. Bandosz P, O'Flaherty M, Drygas W, et al. Decline in mortality from coronary heart disease in Poland after socioeconomic transformation: modelling study. BMJ 2012;344:d8136.
2. Ford ES, Ajani UA, Croft JB, et al. Explaining the decrease in U.S. deaths from coronary disease, 1980-2000. N Engl J Med 2007;356:2388–98.
3. O'Flaherty M, Ford E, Allender S, et al. Coronary heart disease trends in England and Wales from 1984 to 2004: concealed levelling of mortality rates among young adults. Heart 2008;94:178–81.
4. Roger VL, Go AS, Lloyd-Jones DM, et al. Executive summary: heart disease and stroke statistics–2012 update: a report from the American Heart Association. Circulation 2012;125:188–97.
5. Vaartjes I, O'Flaherty M, Grobbee DE, et al. Coronary heart disease mortality trends in the Netherlands 1972-2007. Heart 2011;97:569–73.
6. Bajekal M, Scholes S, Love H, et al. Analysing recent socioeconomic trends in coronary heart disease mortality in England, 2000-2007: a population modelling study. PLoS Med 2012;9:e1001237.
7. Mortality in treated heterozygous familial hypercholesterolaemia: implications for clinical management. Scientific Steering Committee on behalf of the Simon Broome Register Group. Atherosclerosis 1999;142:105–12.
8. Risk of fatal coronary heart disease in familial hypercholesterolaemia. Scientific Steering Committee on behalf of the Simon Broome Register Group. BMJ 1991; 303:893–6.
9. Marks D, Wonderling D, Thorogood M, et al. Screening for hypercholesterolaemia versus case finding for familial hypercholesterolaemia: a systematic review and cost-effectiveness analysis. Health Technol Assess 2000;4:1–123.
10. Brown MS, Goldstein JL. Familial hypercholesterolemia: a genetic defect in the low-density lipoprotein receptor. N Engl J Med 1976;294:1386–90.
11. Talmud PJ, Futema M, Humphries SE. The genetic architecture of the familial hyperlipidaemia syndromes: rare mutations and common variants in multiple genes. Curr Opin Lipidol 2014;25:274–81.
12. Cortner JA, Coates PM, Gallagher PR. Prevalence and expression of familial combined hyperlipidemia in childhood. J Pediatr 1990;116:514–9.
13. Johansen CT, Hegele RA. Genetic bases of hypertriglyceridemic phenotypes. Curr Opin Lipidol 2011;22:247–53.
14. Johansen CT, Kathiresan S, Hegele RA. Genetic determinants of plasma triglycerides. J Lipid Res 2011;52:189–206.
15. Brunzell JD, Iverius PH, Scheibel MS, et al. Primary lipoprotein lipase deficiency. Adv Exp Med Biol 1986;201:227–39.

16. Evans V, Kastelein JJ. Lipoprotein lipase deficiency–rare or common? Cardiovasc Drugs Ther 2002;16:283–7.

17. Miller M, Stone NJ, Ballantyne C, et al. Triglycerides and cardiovascular disease: a scientific statement from the American Heart Association. Circulation 2011;123:2292–333.

18. Cohen JC, Boerwinkle E, Mosley TH Jr, et al. Sequence variations in PCSK9, low LDL, and protection against coronary heart disease. N Engl J Med 2006;354:1264–72.

19. Expert panel on integrated guidelines for cardiovascular health and risk reduction in children and adolescents: summary report. Pediatrics 2011;128(Suppl 5):S213–56.

20. Weintraub WS, Daniels SR, Burke LE, et al. Value of primordial and primary prevention for cardiovascular disease: a policy statement from the American Heart Association. Circulation 2011;124:967–90.

21. Strasser T. Reflections on cardiovascular diseases. Interdiscip Sci Rev 1978;3:225–30.

22. Lewington S, Clarke R, Qizilbash N, et al. Age-specific relevance of usual blood pressure to vascular mortality: a meta-analysis of individual data for one million adults in 61 prospective studies. Lancet 2002;360:1903–13.

23. Di Angelantonio E, Sarwar N, Perry P, et al. Major lipids, apolipoproteins, and risk of vascular disease. JAMA 2009;302:1993–2000.

24. Berenson GS, Srinivasan SR, Bao W, et al. Association between multiple cardiovascular risk factors and atherosclerosis in children and young adults. The Bogalusa Heart Study. N Engl J Med 1998;338:1650–6.

25. Newman WP 3rd, Freedman DS, Voors AW, et al. Relation of serum lipoprotein levels and systolic blood pressure to early atherosclerosis. The Bogalusa Heart Study. N Engl J Med 1986;314:138–44.

26. Natural history of aortic and coronary atherosclerotic lesions in youth. Findings from the PDAY Study. Pathobiological Determinants of Atherosclerosis in Youth (PDAY) Research Group. Arterioscler Thromb 1993;13:1291–8.

27. Rose G. Sick individuals and sick populations. Int J Epidemiol 1985;14:32–8.

28. May AL, Kuklina EV, Yoon PW. Prevalence of cardiovascular disease risk factors among US adolescents, 1999-2008. Pediatrics 2012;129(6):1035–41.

29. The fourth report on the diagnosis, evaluation, and treatment of high blood pressure in children and adolescents. Pediatrics 2004;114:555–76.

30. Daniels SR, Greer FR. Lipid screening and cardiovascular health in childhood. Pediatrics 2008;122:198–208.

31. Dobson AJ, Evans A, Ferrario M, et al. Changes in estimated coronary risk in the 1980s: data from 38 populations in the WHO MONICA project. World Health Organization. Monitoring trends and determinants in cardiovascular diseases. Ann Med 1998;30:199–205.

32. Kuulasmaa K, Tunstall-Pedoe H, Dobson A, et al. Estimation of contribution of changes in classic risk factors to trends in coronary-event rates across the WHO MONICA Project populations. Lancet 2000;355:675–87.

33. Yusuf S, Hawken S, Ounpuu S, et al. Effect of potentially modifiable risk factors associated with myocardial infarction in 52 countries (the INTERHEART study): case-control study. Lancet 2004;364:937–52.

34. O'Donnell MJ, Xavier D, Liu L, et al. Risk factors for ischaemic and intracerebral haemorrhagic stroke in 22 countries (the INTERSTROKE study): a case-control study. Lancet 2010;376:112–23.

35. Gregg EW, Cheng YJ, Cadwell BL, et al. Secular trends in cardiovascular disease risk factors according to body mass index in US adults. JAMA 2005; 293:1868–74.
36. Kit BK, Carroll MD, Lacher DA, et al. Trends in serum lipids among US youths aged 6 to 19 years, 1988-2010. JAMA 2012;308:591–600.
37. Boden WE, O'Rourke RA, Teo KK, et al. Optimal medical therapy with or without PCI for stable coronary disease. N Engl J Med 2007;356:1503–16.
38. Frye RL, August P, Brooks MM, et al. A randomized trial of therapies for type 2 diabetes and coronary artery disease. N Engl J Med 2009;360:2503–15.
39. Velazquez EJ, Lee KL, Deja MA, et al. Coronary-artery bypass surgery in patients with left ventricular dysfunction. N Engl J Med 2011;364:1607–16.
40. Finucane MM, Stevens GA, Cowan MJ, et al. National, regional, and global trends in body-mass index since 1980: systematic analysis of health examination surveys and epidemiological studies with 960 country-years and 9.1 million participants. Lancet 2011;377:557–67.
41. Farzadfar F, Finucane MM, Danaei G, et al. National, regional, and global trends in serum total cholesterol since 1980: systematic analysis of health examination surveys and epidemiological studies with 321 country-years and 3.0 million participants. Lancet 2011;377:578–86.
42. Magnussen CG, Koskinen J, Chen W, et al. Pediatric metabolic syndrome predicts adulthood metabolic syndrome, subclinical atherosclerosis, and type 2 diabetes mellitus but is no better than body mass index alone: the Bogalusa Heart Study and the Cardiovascular Risk in Young Finns Study. Circulation 2010;122:1604–11.
43. Magnussen CG, Raitakari OT, Thomson R, et al. Utility of currently recommended pediatric dyslipidemia classifications in predicting dyslipidemia in adulthood: evidence from the Childhood Determinants of Adult Health (CDAH) study, Cardiovascular Risk in Young Finns study, and Bogalusa Heart Study. Circulation 2008;117:32–42.
44. Gray L, Lee IM, Sesso HD, et al. Blood pressure in early adulthood, hypertension in middle age, and future cardiovascular disease mortality: HAHS (Harvard Alumni Health Study). J Am Coll Cardiol 2011;58:2396–403.
45. Franks PW, Hanson RL, Knowler WC, et al. Childhood obesity, other cardiovascular risk factors, and premature death. N Engl J Med 2010;362:485–93.
46. Koivistoinen T, Hutri-Kahonen N, Juonala M, et al. Metabolic syndrome in childhood and increased arterial stiffness in adulthood: the Cardiovascular Risk in Young Finns study. Ann Med 2011;43:312–9.
47. Avis HJ, Vissers MN, Stein EA, et al. A systematic review and meta-analysis of statin therapy in children with familial hypercholesterolemia. Arterioscler Thromb Vasc Biol 2007;27:1803–10.
48. Carreau V, Girardet JP, Bruckert E. Long-term follow-up of statin treatment in a cohort of children with familial hypercholesterolemia: efficacy and tolerability. Paediatr Drugs 2011;13:267–75.
49. O'Gorman CS, Higgins MF, O'Neill MB. Systematic review and metaanalysis of statins for heterozygous familial hypercholesterolemia in children: evaluation of cholesterol changes and side effects. Pediatr Cardiol 2009;30:482–9.
50. Vuorio A, Kuoppala J, Kovanen PT, et al. Statins for children with familial hypercholesterolemia. Cochrane Database Syst Rev 2010;7:CD006401.
51. Ference BA, Yoo W, Alesh I, et al. Effect of long-term exposure to lower low-density lipoprotein cholesterol beginning early in life on the risk of coronary heart disease: a mendelian randomization analysis. J Am Coll Cardiol 2012;60:2631–9.

52. Wilson JG, Junger G. Principles and practice of screening for disease. In: WHO public health papers no 34. Geneva (Switzerland): World Health Organization; 1968.
53. Stone NJ, Levy RI, Fredrickson DS, et al. Coronary artery disease in 116 kindred with familial type II hyperlipoproteinemia. Circulation 1974;49:476–88.
54. Claassen L, Henneman L, Kindt I, et al. Perceived risk and representations of cardiovascular disease and preventive behaviour in people diagnosed with familial hypercholesterolemia: a cross-sectional questionnaire study. J Health Psychol 2010;15:33–43.
55. Resnicow K, Cross D. Are parents' self-reported total cholesterol levels useful in identifying children with hyperlipidemia? An examination of current guidelines. Pediatrics 1993;92:347–53.
56. Wald DS, Bestwick JP, Wald NJ. Child-parent screening for familial hypercholesterolaemia: screening strategy based on a meta-analysis. BMJ 2007;335:599.
57. Wald DS, Kasturiratne A, Godoy A, et al. Child-parent screening for familial hypercholesterolemia. J Pediatr 2011;159:865–7.
58. Gillman MW, Daniels SR. Is universal pediatric lipid screening justified? JAMA 2012;307:259–60.
59. Klass P. Screening children for cholesterol. In: The New York Times. New York: The New York Times Company; 2012.
60. Newman TB, Pletcher MJ, Hulley SB. Overly aggressive new guidelines for lipid screening in children: evidence of a broken process. Pediatrics 2012;130:349–52.
61. Wang YC, Cheung AM, Bibbins-Domingo K, et al. Effectiveness and cost-effectiveness of blood pressure screening in adolescents in the United States. J Pediatr 2011;158:257–64.e1–7.
62. Ebbeling CB, Leidig MM, Feldman HA, et al. Effects of a low-glycemic load vs low-fat diet in obese young adults: a randomized trial. JAMA 2007;297:2092–102.
63. Jacobson MS, Tomopoulos S, Williams CL, et al. Normal growth in high-risk hyperlipidemic children and adolescents with dietary intervention. Prev Med 1998;27:775–80.
64. Starc TJ, Shea S, Cohn LC, et al. Greater dietary intake of simple carbohydrate is associated with lower concentrations of high-density-lipoprotein cholesterol in hypercholesterolemic children. Am J Clin Nutr 1998;67:1147–54.
65. Van Horn L, Obarzanek E, Barton BA, et al. A summary of results of the Dietary Intervention Study in Children (DISC): lessons learned. Prog Cardiovasc Nurs 2003;18:28–41.
66. Lasky T. Statin use in children in the United States. Pediatrics 2008;122:1406–8.
67. Liberman JN, Berger JE, Lewis M. Prevalence of antihypertensive, antidiabetic, and dyslipidemic prescription medication use among children and adolescents. Arch Pediatr Adolesc Med 2009;163:357–64.
68. Williams RR, Hasstedt SJ, Wilson DE, et al. Evidence that men with familial hypercholesterolemia can avoid early coronary death. An analysis of 77 gene carriers in four Utah pedigrees. JAMA 1986;255:219–24.
69. Keys A, Menotti A, Aravanis C, et al. The seven countries study: 2,289 deaths in 15 years. Prev Med 1984;13:141–54.
70. O'Keefe JH Jr, Cordain L, Harris WH, et al. Optimal low-density lipoprotein is 50 to 70 mg/dl: lower is better and physiologically normal. J Am Coll Cardiol 2004;43:2142–6.
71. Bulbulia R, Bowman L, Wallendszus K, et al. Effects on 11-year mortality and morbidity of lowering LDL cholesterol with simvastatin for about 5 years in 20,536 high-risk individuals: a randomised controlled trial. Lancet 2011;378:2013–20.

Combination Therapy with Statins: Who Benefits?

Amita Singh, MD, Michael Davidson, MD*

KEYWORDS

- Lipids • Cholesterol • Statin • Niacin • Fibrates • Ezetimibe • Omega-3 fatty acids
- Cardiovascular risk

KEY POINTS

- When therapies have been studied in addition to statins, which remain the standard of treatment, it has been challenging to consistently show an additional clinical benefit in terms of cardiovascular (CV) event reduction, although overall safety seems acceptable.
- Combination therapy is a viable and often used strategy, which allows more patients to successfully reach their ideal lipid targets.
- There may be particular benefit with fenofibrate and niacin in patients with more severe atherogenic dyslipidemias who are unable to achieve intensive low-density lipoprotein (LDL) reduction with statins alone.
- Patients with very high CV risk because of recurrent events on therapy, or those with statin intolerance, are potential candidates for combination strategies.
- Further testing of novel therapies, particularly the PCSK9 class of medications, may introduce an era of potent LDL lowering without dependence on statins, but until then, they remain the mainstay of therapy.

INTRODUCTION

Cardiovascular (CV) disease (CVD) has been the leading cause of death in the United States since the early twentieth century, with worldwide rates similarly on the increase.[1] Increased low-density lipoprotein cholesterol (LDL-C) and, to a lesser extent, low high-density lipoprotein cholesterol (HDL-C) and increased triglyceride (TG) levels are all independent risk factors for CVD. Since the introduction of lovastatin in 1987, statins (hemoglobin [HMG]-coenzyme A [CoA] reductase inhibitors) have been repeatedly shown to decrease LDL-C, thereby reducing the risk for CVD events for patients with or without established vascular disease, and have long comprised the foundation of lipid-lowering therapy.

The importance of decreasing LDL levels in modification of CV risk has driven interest in and development of several novel cholesterol-modifying drugs, many of

Section of Cardiology, University of Chicago, Chicago, IL, USA
* Corresponding author. 140 Belle Avenue, Highland Park, IL 60035.
E-mail address: mdavidsonmd@gmail.com

Endocrinol Metab Clin N Am 43 (2014) 993–1006
http://dx.doi.org/10.1016/j.ecl.2014.08.005

endo.theclinics.com

which are under investigation in ongoing clinical trials. However, until these pharmacotherapies are widely available, the established cholesterol-modifying drugs remain the cornerstone of therapy; among these are statins, niacin, fibrates, ezetimibe, bile acid sequestrants (BASs), and omega-3 fatty acids (OM3FAs). In the last 10 years, clinical trials of combination therapy, primarily used as add-on therapies to statins, have yielded inconsistent results with regards to CV-related morbidity and mortality outcomes. Further complicating the picture are the release of the 2013 American College of Cardiology (ACC)/American Heart Association (AHA) Guidelines on the Treatment of Blood Cholesterol, which shifted the focus of therapy away from LDL-C targets.[2] The juxtaposition of these guidelines with previous algorithms has invoked questions regarding the safety and efficacy of combination lipid-lowering therapies as part of an optimal medical regimen for CV risk reduction. Although combination therapy may not be broadly recommended for all patients, closer examination of the available data suggests that combination therapy is largely safe and that careful selection provides tailored lipid-lowering strategies, which may benefit specific populations.

QUESTIONING THE PARADIGM: UPDATED BLOOD CHOLESTEROL GUIDELINES

Until recently, the aim of lipid-lowering therapy had focused on an established LDL-C target, which was calculated based on the presence of CV risk factors or equivalent disease states. In turn, this risk estimate and target LDL-C mandated how medication therapies were initiated and further titrated, typically beginning with statins.[3] The National Cholesterol Education Panel delineated LDL-C as the primary target of statin therapy, with a secondary non–HDL-C goal (designated as 30 mg/dL more than the LDL-C target). Intensive therapy was geared toward patients with higher risk, as assessed by the 10-year risk estimates using the Framingham scoring system, with consideration for use of add-on therapies for achievement of LDL-C or non–HDL-C targets. Commonly cited weaknesses of the 2001 guidelines and 2004 update were the limited generalizability of the Framingham risk score in women and nonwhite populations, and the monolithic emphasis on LDL-C targets, which could possibly lead to underuse of statin therapy. Efforts to expound on these guidelines emerged from consensus statements and guidelines from the American Diabetes Association and AHA/ACC, which further elaborated on the identification of high-risk patients (so-called cardiometabolic patients and those with established CVD), for whom intensive lipid-lowering therapy would provide incremental benefit in residual CV risk reduction.[4–6]

In a hotly debated turn, the 2013 ACC/AHA Guidelines on the Treatment of Blood Cholesterol abandoned the prespecified LDL-C and non–HDL-C targets in favor of the identification of 4 risk groups for whom statin therapy is most likely to be beneficial in reducing the risk of atherosclerotic CVD.[2] Furthermore, in lieu of designated on-treatment LDL-C targets, the guidelines suggested an empirical statin potency (low, mid, or high potency) without clear targets. It can be surmised that assessing a response to therapy (ie, percent LDL reduction) could be obtained from measuring on-treatment lipid values, although the panel did not recommend routine pursuit of LDL-C targets. The 2013 guidelines do not discuss details of combination therapy, although it is implied that there may be a role for add-on strategies in individuals with statin intolerance or those with a suboptimal response to therapy. Thus, the guideline-driven use of combination therapy in the era of statin therapy remains open ended, with answers likely to be clarified by the results of future clinical trials.

STATINS AS FIRST-LINE THERAPY

The largest and most convincing body of clinical trial–based evidence supporting reduction in CV outcomes with lipid-lowering therapies is ascribed to the statin class of drugs. Statins act as competitive inhibitors with HMG-CoA reductase, an enzyme critical to the rate-limiting step in the biosynthesis of cholesterol, because it catalyzes the conversion of HMG-CoA to mevalonic acid. The downstream effects of reduced cholesterol synthesis lead to upregulation of LDL receptors and increased plasma clearance of LDL-C. Lipid-independent pleiotropic effects of statins include improved endothelial function via activation of eNOS, reduction of circulating oxidized lipoproteins, and antiinflammatory effects via suppressed production of proinflammatory cytokines.[7] Imaging studies including intravascular ultrasonography and magnetic resonance imaging modalities have suggested the stabilizing effects of statin therapy on plaque composition by showing plaque lipid depletion and even regression in limited studies.[8–10]

Primary prevention studies of statin therapy have shown benefits through reduction of LDL-C levels along with subsequent decreases in the incidence of coronary disease events in numerous populations, including diabetics (CARDS [Collaborative Atorvastatin Diabetes Study]), the elderly (PROSPER), hypertensive patients (ASCOT-BPLA), and those with high LDL-C levels (WOSCOPS, AFCAPS/Tex-CAPS [Air Force/Texas Coronary Atherosclerosis Prevention Study]).[11–17] Furthermore, an increasing body of evidence suggests that individuals with baseline evidence of increased inflammation, manifest as increases in high-sensitivity C-reactive protein, may experience an even greater benefit of statins mediated through both LDL-lowering and antiinflammatory effects.[18–21] Secondary prevention studies have not only shown a reduction in recurrent CV events with statin therapy for patients with established vascular disease but also a reduction in mortality.[22–27] Data from more recent clinical trials and meta-analyses[22,27,28] have underscored the observation that further LDL-C lowering may be of additional benefit in a very high-risk secondary prevention population. Furthermore, the benefits gleaned from statin use may be continuous over decreasing levels of LDL. An estimated 10% to 12% reduction in all-cause mortality, driven by CV-related mortality, accompanies each 1-mmol/L reduction of LDL-C, which supported the pursuit of more intensive LDL-C goals for certain high-risk populations.[23,29]

LIMITATIONS OF STATIN MONOTHERAPY

Ideally, combining another drug with a statin would improve on CV risk reduction and lessen the likelihood of adverse side effects. Although statins are clearly beneficial, they can be associated with clinically significant adverse reactions and side effects, which may impair adherence or prevent optimal titration. The incidence of musculoskeletal-related issues, most commonly myalgias, was reported in only 1.5% to 5% of patients in clinical trials, whereas observational studies in general statin-treated populations have reported significantly higher rates of up to 10%.[30,31] More serious side effects include myopathy, defined as increased creatine phosphokinase level 10 times the upper limit of normal, and rhabdomyolysis (myopathy with concomitant renal injury), although both entities are less common. Predisposing patient factors associated with a greater incidence of myopathy include elderly age, female gender, renal impairment, hypothyroidism, and the use of interacting drugs (eg, CYP3A4 or CYP2C9 substrates).[32] Statins have also been shown to potentially increase aminotransferase levels, although this may be dose related and also associated with underlying nonalcoholic hepatic steatosis, which improves with therapy.

Overt hepatotoxicity is rare, but caution should be advised for patients with a history of liver dysfunction.[33] Recent attention has been drawn to the potential unmasking of incident diabetes with statin use. This situation seems to be more pronounced with intensive-dose compared with moderate-dose statins, although the risk is outweighed by the magnitude of CV risk reduction seen with their use.[34]

Although statin therapy results in significant reductions in LDL-C levels, it does not affect all components of the lipid profile equally. In cardiometabolic patients with atherogenic dyslipidemia, manifest as increased TG and low HDL-C levels, there may be a role for combination therapy. Post hoc analyses of intensive statin therapy have suggested that persistently increases apolipoprotein B (ApoB) and TG levels are associated with recurrent CV events, reinforcing the concept that although statins are part of optimal medical therapy, they do not entirely mitigate residual risk.[35,36] Therefore, add-on therapies may be appropriate for patients with increased TG or ApoB levels, in addition to those who experience recurrent events on statin therapy.

Strategies for Combination Therapy: Safety and Efficacy

Niacin and statin combination therapy

Niacin is one of the oldest lipid-lowering drugs in active use, and acts to lower LDL-C levels through several mechanisms, including limiting peripheral mobilization of free fatty acids, thereby limiting hepatic very low-density lipoprotein (VLDL) synthesis, as well as interfering with the conversion of VLDL to LDL-C. It results in dose-dependent reductions in LDL-C of up to 15%, and at lower doses, can improve HDL-C by 15% to 40%, and lower TG levels by 25% to 50%. Some of the earliest data using niacin monotherapy in men with previous myocardial infarction (MI) showed a durable CV morbidity and mortality benefit gained with administration of niacin at 3 g per day.[37,38] Additional data gleaned from combination niacin-statin trials using surrogate measures of atherosclerosis, as in the HATS (HDL Atherosclerosis Treatment Study) and ARBITER-3 studies, suggested a possible regression in coronary stenosis and carotid intima-medial thickness, respectively, with combination therapy.[39,40] There are concerns related to its number of side effects, which include flushing, hepatotoxicity, worsening of impaired glucose tolerance, and hyperuricemia.

Recent larger-scale clinical trials of niacin as add-on therapy to statins have yielded less convincing results in altering CVD events. Results from AIM-HIGH (Atherothrombosis Intervention in Metabolic Syndrome with Low HDL/High Triglycerides: Impact on Global Health Outcomes) were released in 2011, because the trial ended earlier than anticipated because of an interim analysis suggesting futility in proving its hypothesis.[41] The study population, comprising patients with atherogenic dyslipidemia and previous CVD, had achieved intensive LDL-C control with combination simvastatin-ezetimibe, with a mean of 71 mg/dL at the start of the trial. Thus, many of these high-risk patients embarked on the trial having already achieved their lipid goals. During the truncated 3-year follow-up period, there was no difference in the composite event of coronary heart disease, nonfatal MI, ischemic stroke, hospitalization for an acute coronary syndrome, or symptom-driven coronary or cerebral revascularization (hazard ratio [HR] 1.02, 95% confidence interval [CI] 0.87–1.21, $P = .79$). Recently published subgroup data posited that there was a trend toward benefit with niacin therapy for patients with the highest tertile of TG (>198 mg/dL) and lowest tertile of HDL-C (<33 mg/dL), although it did not meet significance (HR 0.74, $P = .073$).[42]

Although formal publications are forthcoming, data are available from the HPS2-THRIVE (Treatment of HDL to Reduce the Incidence of Vascular Events) trial, in which niacin-laropiprant versus placebo was tested against a background therapy for simvastatin-ezetimibe and failed to prove benefit in rates of major vascular events (relative risk [RR] 0.96, 95% CI 0.90–1.03, $P = .29$) over 4 years of follow-up.[43] Furthermore, safety end points from the trial raised concerns because of a signal for increased hemorrhagic stroke rates associated with treatment, although the trend toward risk with niacin-laropiprant therapy was not significant (RR 1.28, 95% CI 0.97–1.69, $P = .08$). The well-publicized increased rates of myopathy (RR 4.4, $P<.0001$), particularly in patients of Chinese descent, were not accompanied by a significant increase in rhabdomyolysis (7 cases in treatment vs 5 in placebo, RR 1.4, $= 0.54$), they still suggested a common reason for drug discontinuation.[44] Subgroup data are yet to be made available from this trial, although there was a hint toward possible benefit for a small subgroup of patients with LDL-C levels more than 77 mg/dL (12% for niacin-laropiprant vs 13.5% for placebo, $P = .02$). Both trials aimed to assess the CV benefits gleaned from primarily HDL increasing, although niacin was shown to lower LDL-C levels in both trials (−12.5% reduction in AIM-HIGH, −10% LDL-C reduction in HPS2-THRIVE) without conferring clear and additional CV risk benefit. A flaw in study design that may have contributed to the failure of either AIM-HIGH or HPS2-THRIVE to prove a significant difference in outcomes relates to the small differences in non–HDL-C between treatment groups at the conclusion of the study. In AIM-HIGH, the non-HDL difference was 101 mg/dL, whereas in HPS2-THRIVE, the non-HDL difference was a mere 17 mg/dL. These small differences may have made it difficult to detect a treatment effect between groups, and helps underscore why there was no improvement in risk detected for these populations who were already on intensive lipid-lowering therapy with statins.

The 2013 ACC/AHA guidelines cite that based on the results of AIM-HIGH, there is no apparent CVD benefit for patients who are at their LDL-C goal (between 40 and 80 mg/dL).[2] Although the 2 trials discussed have weakened the strength of evidence supporting the use of niacin, it remains an effective LDL-lowering agent and should be considered as a combination strategy, particularly for patients who have combined increased TG and LDL-C levels without contraindications for its use.

Statins and fibrate combination therapy

Fibric acid derivatives exert a primarily TG-lowering effect via activation of the α subtype of the peroxisome proliferator-activated receptor (PPAR-α), a nuclear hormone receptor. Stimulation of PPAR-α increases lipolysis through simultaneous upregulation of LPL, thereby increasing VLDL catabolism and TG clearance from plasma, but can also lead to small increases in LDL in patients with baseline increased TG levels.

Although fibrates are used in conjunction with statin therapy, their lipid-lowering effects extend beyond reductions in LDL-C ($\leq$10%–20%, again primarily in patients without increased TG levels), because they have also been shown to lower TG levels up to 20% to 50% and increase HDL-C by 5% to 15%.[45] Gemfibrozil is a first-generation fibric acid derivative, and was shown in VA-HIT (Veterans Affairs HDL Intervention Trial)[46] to reduce nonfatal MI and CV death by 4.4% (RR reduction [RRR] of 22%, $P = .006$) when used in dyslipidemic men with previous coronary artery disease compared with the placebo group, despite similarly achieved LDL-C levels. There was an even greater benefit seen for patients with diabetes mellitus or those with increasing plasma insulin levels without overt diabetes.[47] However, gemfibrozil acts by inhibiting hepatic glucuronidation and may potentiate circulating levels of statin, potentially leading to greater risk of toxicity in combination therapy.

Newer formulations, particularly fenofibrate, have been shown to have a lower toxicity profile. This finding was verified in a pooled analysis of 6 clinical trials[48] evaluating coadministration of fenofibrate with statins, in which there were no significant differences in overall adverse events compared with statin monotherapy, including no reports of myopathy or rhabdomyolysis in the 1628 subjects studied. Although the fenofibrate-statin combination fares better in safety data, there is inconsistent evidence for their use to modify CV outcomes. The well-publicized results from the ACCORD (Lipid-lowering Action to Control Cardiovascular Risk in Diabetes) trial,[49] which pitted combination simvastatin-fenofibrate versus simvastatin alone in a diabetic population, failed to show any reduction in the primary composite end point over 4.7 years of follow-up, despite improvements in TG and HDL-C levels in the combination arm. However, an important subgroup emerged, in whom the combination of fenofibrate-simvastatin did confer benefit; although the overall cohort had a nonsignificant RRR in the primary outcome of 8%, patients with TG levels greater than 204 mg/dL and HDL-C levels less than 34 mg/dL had a trend toward a greater RRR (–31%, P = .057). Review of data from older fibrate monotherapy studies (FIELD, HHS, BIP)[50] similarly seem to point to this low–HDL-C/high-TG group as one that experiences the greatest degree of benefit with the use of fibrate therapy.

Furthermore, the safety of this combination seems to have been borne out in trials using fenofibrate. In ACCORD, there was no significant difference in rates of myopathy or increases in creatine phosphokinase levels, again suggesting that the combination of fenofibrate with simvastatin was well tolerated. Although the FIELD trial was intended to analyze the benefit of fibrate monotherapy, nearly one-third of patients in the fibrate arm were initiated on statin therapy, and of those nearly 1000 patients, there were no reported cases of rhabdomyolysis.[51]

A meta-analysis of 18 trials[52] including more than 45,000 patients found that there was no significant mortality benefit with fibrate therapy, but a 10% RRR (P = .048) for overall CV events and 13% RRR for coronary events (P<.001). Taken together, these data suggest that fibrates are not routinely indicated second-line therapy for LDL lowering, nor do they alter mortality outcomes, but their use may result in CV and coronary event reduction for patients with diabetes and an atherogenic dyslipidemic lipid profile.

Bile acid sequestrant and statin combination therapy

Before the advent of statins, BAS therapy with either cholestyramine or colestipol was proved to be an effective LDL-C–lowering strategy, with early data showing associated reductions in coronary heart disease (CHD) event rates compared with placebo.[53–55] In conjunction with statin therapy, BAS can provide an additive reduction in LDL-C levels by 10% to 25%. A caveat for their use relates to a potential increase in TG level for patients with baseline hypertriglyceridemia, which may be related to a compensatory increase in VLDL production. In addition, the use of BAS as part of a combination therapy is limited by their interference with statin absorption, potentially leading to decreased efficacy of therapy.[56]

The emergence of a second-generation BAS, colesevelam, has largely circumvented the drug-drug interactions that marred the use of older-generation BAS. Colesevelam is further appealing among the BAS class because of added improvements in HDL-C and ApoB in combination with atorvastatin.[57] An intriguing glucose-lowering effect of colesevelam was shown in the GLOWS (Glucose Lowering Effect of WelChol Study), in which a small population of diabetic patients were randomized to colesevelam 3.65 g/d versus placebo for 12 weeks, at which time there was a significant reduction in A1c by –0.5% (up to –1.0% for those with baseline HbA1c >8.0%) and reductions in LDL-C (–11.7% treatment difference), as well as ApoB and LDL particle number.[58] Thus, there may be a role for add-on BAS therapy to statins, namely colesevelam, in patients with type 2 diabetes mellitus, although caution must be exercised to avoid its use in patients with hypertriglyceridemia.

Ezetimibe and statin combination therapy

Ezetimibe is a cholesterol absorption inhibitor that works at the level of the Niemann-Pick C1-like 1 protein in the small bowel, capable of decreasing LDL-C levels by up to 20% when used in conjunction with statins.[59–61] Use of ezetimibe as add-on therapy reduces circulating levels of proinflammatory oxidized LDL-C and LDL particle number.[62,63]

Despite the contemporary use of ezetimibe, there are only a few clinical trials that have examined its use within specific patient populations. A secondary analysis from SANDS (Stop Atherosclerosis in Native Diabetics Study)[64] showed regression in carotid intima-medial thickness in diabetics treated to aggressive LDL-C targets regardless of treatment (statin monotherapy vs combination with ezetimibe), indicating that although it was an effective strategy to achieve LDL lowering, there was no treatment-independent benefit gained from its use. The SHARP (Study of Heart and Renal Protection) trial[60] randomized 9270 patients with renal disease to simvastatin-ezetimibe versus placebo, with a significant reduction seen in the primary end point of coronary death, nonfatal MI, stroke, or revascularization (13.4% vs 11.3%, $P = .002$). Evidence of a reduction in CV events within the population with renal disease is particularly notable, because previous statin trials had not been able to replicate a magnitude of benefit. Another study comparing simvastatin-ezetimibe with placebo in patients with mild to moderate aortic stenosis (SEAS [Simvastatin and Ezetimibe in Aortic Stenosis])[59] did not show a reduction in the primary outcome of valvular and ischemic events, but there was a significant reduction in ischemic events by 22%, which was a prespecified secondary outcome. The most common side effects of combination statin-ezetimibe related to transaminase abnormalities, with 1 pooled analysis of safety outcomes[65] estimating an overall incidence less than 1%, consistent with what is reported in the prescribing information.

Benefits of ezetimibe use are extrapolated from the limited series of studies as outlined earlier. IMPROVE-IT (Improved Reduction of Outcomes: Vytorin Efficacy International Trial), which is assessing the use of simvastatin-ezetimibe versus simvastatin in a post-ACS population, should be completed soon and will no doubt enrich the current body of evidence on add-on ezetimibe use.[66]

Omega-3 fatty acids and statin combination therapy

OM3FAs, namely docosahexaenoic acid (DHA) and eicosapentanoic acid (EPA), have been shown to reduce TG levels in a dose-dependent fashion, with largely neutral effects on LDL-C. Earlier secondary prevention studies[67,68] suggested that supplementation with low-dose daily OM3FAs resulted in 15% to 20% reduction in composite CV events for patients with and without a history of coronary artery disease. Subsequent prospective studies[69–71] performed in the era of high-potency statins have failed to replicate these findings. This finding is well illustrated by results from the Alpha Omega trial,[72] which examined the outcomes of low-dose supplementation EPA+DHA in a secondary prevention setting in conjunction with modern medical therapy, with 86% of patients enrolled receiving statin therapy. The negative results for the overall study population suggested that there was a significant interaction in treatment effect seen in patients who were treated with statins, although post hoc analyses did suggest significant benefit for diabetic patients with history of an MI and for patients who were not on statin therapy. The doses of omega-3s used in these trials were ineffective in lowering TGs and therefore may have been inadequate to provide a lipid benefit necessary to reduce CHD events.

Newer formulations of OM3FA (Vascepa, Epanova), highly refined to allow for higher potency of EPA or EPA+DHA, have been shown to effectively treat hypertriglyceridemia and seem to have non–HDL-C–lowering effects, which may be augmented by concomitant high-potency statin use.[73–76] In addition, the combination of statins and OM3FAs seem to be safe and well tolerated, with the most frequent side effect of gastrointestinal intolerance. However, there are no definitive data to suggest a further reduction of CV events with the use of these newer OM3FA formulations. Ongoing clinical trials (REDUCE-IT, STRENGTH) will aim to answer whether the benefits of OM3FA with statin therapy extend beyond TG level lowering to confer any primary or secondary CV RR in patients with hypertriglyceridemia on statin therapy.

Novel Add-On Therapies

Mipomersen and lomitapide are both therapies approved by the US Food and Drug Administration for use as adjunctive to maximally tolerated lipid-lowering medications and diet, specifically for the treatment of homozygous familial hypercholesterolemia (FH). Mipomersen is an apoB-100 antisense oligonucleotide, administered as a subcutaneous injection, which binds to ApoB messenger RNA and curtails hepatic synthesis of ApoB-containing lipoproteins.[77] Main side effects relate to increased liver transaminase levels, injection site reactions, and systemic symptoms of fatigue and pyrexia. Lomitapide is an inhibitor of microsomal TG transfer protein and decreases LDL as well as TG levels.[77] The primary side effect relates to gastrointestinal side effects, and more serious complications related to hepatotoxicity and fatty liver, and have led to limiting prescribing under terms of Risk Evaluation and Mitigation Strategy in the United States.

The promise of PCSK-9 inhibitors, which targets the enzyme that regulates LDL-receptor degradation to promote receptor-mediated clearance of LDL from plasma, only continues to grow with accumulating phase 2 and phase 3 clinical trials. Various antibody formulations have been shown to result in marked LDL-C reductions in FH and the statin-intolerant population, and preliminary data suggest safety and sustained efficacy when used in conjunction with statin therapy with up to 1 year of treatment. Reductions have been dramatic, with 49% to 76% decreases in LDL-C levels as part of monotherapy or used alongside either high-potency statins or daily ezetimibe.[78–83] This striking potency in lipid lowering has allowed greater numbers of at-risk patients to achieve ideal LDL-C targets, which may be difficult for patients with FH or intensive goals of less than 70 mg/dL.[84,85] Concurrent reductions in ApoB, Lp(a), TG, VLDL, and modest increases in HDL-C levels have all been reported, further reinforcing their appeal for clinical use. However, when and for whom this class of medications will be approved and adopted for widespread use will depend on the ease of their required subcutaneous administration routes and durable safety data, which are still undergoing longer-term investigation.

SUMMARY

Individually, many of the lipid-lowering drugs in use have been shown to improve CV outcomes. However, when therapies have been studied in addition to statins, which remain the standard of treatment, it has been challenging to consistently show an additional clinical benefit in terms of CV event reduction, although overall safety seems acceptable. This debate has been further complicated by the advent of recent guidelines, which emphasize treatment with high-potency statin monotherapy over achievement of discrete LDL-C and non–HDL-C targets. Combination therapy is a viable and often used strategy that allows more patients to successfully reach their ideal lipid targets. There may be particular benefit with fenofibrate and niacin in patients with more severe atherogenic dyslipidemias who are unable to achieve intensive LDL reduction with statins alone. In addition, patients with very high CV risk because of recurrent events on therapy, or those with statin intolerance, are potential candidates for combination strategies. Further testing of novel therapies, particularly the PCSK-9 class of medications, may introduce an era of potent LDL lowering without dependence on statins, but until then, they remain the mainstay of therapy.

REFERENCES

1. Fuster V, Kelly BB, editors. Promoting cardiovascular health in the developing world: a critical challenge to achieve global health. Washington, DC: 2010.
2. Stone NJ. 2013 ACC/AHA guideline on the treatment of blood cholesterol to reduce atherosclerotic cardiovascular risk in adults: a report of the American College of Cardiology/American Heart Association Task Force on Practice Guidelines. J Am Coll Cardiol 2013;63(25 Pt B):2889–934.
3. National Cholesterol Education Program (NCEP) Expert Panel on Detection, Evaluation, and Treatment of High Blood Cholesterol in Adults (Adult Treatment Panel III). Third Report of the National Cholesterol Education Program (NCEP) Expert Panel on Detection, Evaluation, and Treatment of High Blood Cholesterol in Adults (Adult Treatment Panel III) final report. Circulation 2002;106(25): 3143–421.
4. American Diabetes Association. Standards of medical care in diabetes–2013. Diabetes Care 2013;36(Suppl 1):S11–66.
5. Brunzell JD. Lipoprotein management in patients with cardiometabolic risk: consensus statement from the American Diabetes Association and the American College of Cardiology Foundation. Diabetes Care 2008;31(4):811–22.
6. AHA. AHA/ACC guidelines for secondary prevention for patients with coronary and other atherosclerotic vascular disease: 2006 update endorsed by the National Heart, Lung, and Blood Institute. J Am Coll Cardiol 2006;47(10):2130–9.
7. Bonetti PO. Statin effects beyond lipid lowering–are they clinically relevant? Eur Heart J 2003;24(3):225–48.
8. Nicholls SJ. Effect of two intensive statin regimens on progression of coronary disease. N Engl J Med 2011;365(22):2078–87.
9. Nissen SE. Effect of very high-intensity statin therapy on regression of coronary atherosclerosis: the ASTEROID trial. JAMA 2006;295(13):1556–65.
10. Zhao XQ. MR imaging of carotid plaque composition during lipid-lowering therapy a prospective assessment of effect and time course. JACC Cardiovasc Imaging 2011;4(9):977–86.
11. Downs JR. Primary prevention of acute coronary events with lovastatin in men and women with average cholesterol levels: results of AFCAPS/TexCAPS. Air Force/Texas Coronary Atherosclerosis Prevention Study. JAMA 1998;279(20): 1615–22.
12. Heart Protection Study Collaborative Group. MRC/BHF Heart Protection Study of cholesterol lowering with simvastatin in 20,536 high-risk individuals: a randomised placebo-controlled trial. Lancet 2002;360(9326):7–22.
13. ALLHAT Officers and Coordinators for the ALLHAT Collaborative Research Group, The Antihypertensive and Lipid-Lowering Treatment to Prevent Heart Attack Trial. Major outcomes in moderately hypercholesterolemic, hypertensive

patients randomized to pravastatin vs usual care: The Antihypertensive and Lipid-Lowering Treatment to Prevent Heart Attack Trial (ALLHAT-LLT). JAMA 2002;288(23):2998–3007.

14. Shepherd J. Prevention of coronary heart disease with pravastatin in men with hypercholesterolemia. West of Scotland Coronary Prevention Study Group. N Engl J Med 1995;333(20):1301–7.

15. Shepherd J. Pravastatin in elderly individuals at risk of vascular disease (PROSPER): a randomised controlled trial. Lancet 2002;360(9346):1623–30.

16. Colhoun HM. Primary prevention of cardiovascular disease with atorvastatin in type 2 diabetes in the Collaborative Atorvastatin Diabetes Study (CARDS): multicentre randomised placebo-controlled trial. Lancet 2004;364(9435): 685–96.

17. Sever PS. Prevention of coronary and stroke events with atorvastatin in hypertensive patients who have average or lower-than-average cholesterol concentrations, in the Anglo-Scandinavian Cardiac Outcomes Trial–Lipid Lowering Arm (ASCOT-LLA): a multicentre randomised controlled trial. Lancet 2003; 361(9364):1149–58.

18. Ridker PM. C-reactive protein levels and outcomes after statin therapy. N Engl J Med 2005;352(1):20–8.

19. Ridker PM. Relative efficacy of atorvastatin 80 mg and pravastatin 40 mg in achieving the dual goals of low-density lipoprotein cholesterol <70 mg/dl and C-reactive protein <2 mg/l: an analysis of the PROVE-IT TIMI-22 trial. J Am Coll Cardiol 2005;45(10):1644–8.

20. Morrow DA. Clinical relevance of C-reactive protein during follow-up of patients with acute coronary syndromes in the Aggrastat-to-Zocor Trial. Circulation 2006; 114(4):281–8.

21. Ridker PM. Rosuvastatin to prevent vascular events in men and women with elevated C-reactive protein. N Engl J Med 2008;359(21):2195–207.

22. LaRosa JC. Intensive lipid lowering with atorvastatin in patients with stable coronary disease. N Engl J Med 2005;352(14):1425–35.

23. Cholesterol Treatment Trialists' (CTT) Collaboration, et al. Efficacy and safety of more intensive lowering of LDL cholesterol: a meta-analysis of data from 170,000 participants in 26 randomised trials. Lancet 2010;376(9753):1670–81.

24. Prevention of cardiovascular events and death with pravastatin in patients with coronary heart disease and a broad range of initial cholesterol levels. The Long-Term Intervention with Pravastatin in Ischaemic Disease (LIPID) Study Group. N Engl J Med 1998;339(19):1349–57.

25. Sacks FM. The effect of pravastatin on coronary events after myocardial infarction in patients with average cholesterol levels. Cholesterol and Recurrent Events Trial investigators. N Engl J Med 1996;335(14):1001–9.

26. Randomised trial of cholesterol lowering in 4444 patients with coronary heart disease: the Scandinavian Simvastatin Survival Study (4S). Lancet 1994; 344(8934):1383–9.

27. Cannon CP. Intensive versus moderate lipid lowering with statins after acute coronary syndromes. N Engl J Med 2004;350(15):1495–504.

28. Pedersen TR. High-dose atorvastatin vs usual-dose simvastatin for secondary prevention after myocardial infarction: the IDEAL study: a randomized controlled trial. JAMA 2005;294(19):2437–45.

29. Baigent C. Efficacy and safety of cholesterol-lowering treatment: prospective meta-analysis of data from 90,056 participants in 14 randomised trials of statins. Lancet 2005;366(9493):1267–78.

30. Bays H. Statin safety: an overview and assessment of the data–2005. Am J Cardiol 2006;97(8A):6C–26C.
31. Bruckert E. Mild to moderate muscular symptoms with high-dosage statin therapy in hyperlipidemic patients–the PRIMO study. Cardiovasc Drugs Ther 2005; 19(6):403–14.
32. Bitzur R. Intolerance to statins: mechanisms and management. Diabetes Care 2013;36(Suppl 2):S325–30.
33. Tandra S, Vuppalanchi R. Use of statins in patients with liver disease. Curr Treat Options Cardiovasc Med 2009;11(4):272–8.
34. Preiss D. Risk of incident diabetes with intensive-dose compared with moderate-dose statin therapy: a meta-analysis. JAMA 2011;305(24):2556–64.
35. Mora S. Determinants of residual risk in secondary prevention patients treated with high- versus low-dose statin therapy: the Treating to New Targets (TNT) study. Circulation 2012;125(16):1979–87.
36. Faergeman O. Plasma triglycerides and cardiovascular events in the Treating to New Targets and Incremental Decrease in End-Points through Aggressive Lipid Lowering trials of statins in patients with coronary artery disease. Am J Cardiol 2009;104(4):459–63.
37. Canner PL. Fifteen year mortality in Coronary Drug Project patients: long-term benefit with niacin. J Am Coll Cardiol 1986;8(6):1245–55.
38. Clofibrate and niacin in coronary heart disease. JAMA 1975;231(4):360–81.
39. Taylor AJ, Lee HJ, Sullenberger LE. The effect of 24 months of combination statin and extended-release niacin on carotid intima-media thickness: ARBITER 3. Curr Med Res Opin 2006;22(11):2243–50.
40. Brown BG. Simvastatin and niacin, antioxidant vitamins, or the combination for the prevention of coronary disease. N Engl J Med 2001;345(22):1583–92.
41. AIM-HIGH Investigators, et al. Niacin in patients with low HDL cholesterol levels receiving intensive statin therapy. N Engl J Med 2011;365(24):2255–67.
42. Guyton JR. Relationship of lipoproteins to cardiovascular events: the AIM-HIGH Trial (Atherothrombosis Intervention in Metabolic Syndrome With Low HDL/High Triglycerides and Impact on Global Health Outcomes). J Am Coll Cardiol 2013; 62(17):1580–4.
43. HPS2-THRIVE: Randomized placebo-controlled trial of ER niacin and laropiprant in 25,673 patients with pre-existing cardiovascular disease. American College of Cardiology Scientific Sessions.
44. HPS2-THRIVE Collaborative Group. HPS2-THRIVE randomized placebo-controlled trial in 25 673 high-risk patients of ER niacin/laropiprant: trial design, pre-specified muscle and liver outcomes, and reasons for stopping study treatment. Eur Heart J 2013;34(17):1279–91.
45. Staels B. Mechanism of action of fibrates on lipid and lipoprotein metabolism. Circulation 1998;98(19):2088–93.
46. Rubins HB. Gemfibrozil for the secondary prevention of coronary heart disease in men with low levels of high-density lipoprotein cholesterol. Veterans Affairs High-Density Lipoprotein Cholesterol Intervention Trial Study Group. N Engl J Med 1999;341(6):410–8.
47. Rubins HB. Diabetes, plasma insulin, and cardiovascular disease: subgroup analysis from the Department of Veterans Affairs high-density lipoprotein intervention trial (VA-HIT). Arch Intern Med 2002;162(22):2597–604.
48. Guo J. Meta-analysis of safety of the coadministration of statin with fenofibrate in patients with combined hyperlipidemia. Am J Cardiol 2012;110(9): 1296–301.

49. ACCORD Study Group. Effects of combination lipid therapy in type 2 diabetes mellitus. N Engl J Med 2010;362(17):1563–74.
50. Singh A. What should we do about hypertriglyceridemia in coronary artery disease patients? Curr Treat Options Cardiovasc Med 2013;15(1):104–17.
51. Keech A, Simes RJ, Barter P. Effects of long-term fenofibrate therapy on cardiovascular events in 9795 people with type 2 diabetes mellitus (the FIELD study): randomised controlled trial. Lancet 2005;366(9500):1849–61.
52. Jun M. Effects of fibrates on cardiovascular outcomes: a systematic review and meta-analysis. Lancet 2010;375(9729):1875–84.
53. Glueck CJ. Colestipol and cholestyramine resin. Comparative effects in familial type II hyperlipoproteinemia. JAMA 1972;222(6):676–81.
54. Hashim SA, Vanitallie TB. Cholestyramine resin therapy for hypercholesteremia: clinical and metabolic studies. JAMA 1965;192:289–93.
55. The Lipid Research Clinics Coronary Primary Prevention Trial results. I. Reduction in incidence of coronary heart disease. JAMA 1984;251(3):351–64.
56. Bellosta S, Paoletti R, Corsini A. Safety of statins: focus on clinical pharmacokinetics and drug interactions. Circulation 2004;109(23 Suppl 1):III50–7.
57. Hunninghake D. Coadministration of colesevelam hydrochloride with atorvastatin lowers LDL cholesterol additively. Atherosclerosis 2001;158(2):407–16.
58. Zieve FJ. Results of the glucose-lowering effect of WelChol study (GLOWS): a randomized, double-blind, placebo-controlled pilot study evaluating the effect of colesevelam hydrochloride on glycemic control in subjects with type 2 diabetes. Clin Ther 2007;29(1):74–83.
59. Rossebo AB. Intensive lipid lowering with simvastatin and ezetimibe in aortic stenosis. N Engl J Med 2008;359(13):1343–56.
60. Baigent C. The effects of lowering LDL cholesterol with simvastatin plus ezetimibe in patients with chronic kidney disease (Study of Heart and Renal Protection): a randomised placebo-controlled trial. Lancet 2011;377(9784):2181–92.
61. Morrone D. Lipid-altering efficacy of ezetimibe plus statin and statin monotherapy and identification of factors associated with treatment response: a pooled analysis of over 21,000 subjects from 27 clinical trials. Atherosclerosis 2012; 223(2):251–61.
62. Moutzouri E. Comparison of the effect of simvastatin versus simvastatin/ezetimibe versus rosuvastatin on markers of inflammation and oxidative stress in subjects with hypercholesterolemia. Atherosclerosis 2013;231(1):8–14.
63. Le NA. Changes in lipoprotein particle number with ezetimibe/simvastatin coadministered with extended-release niacin in hyperlipidemic patients. J Am Heart Assoc 2013;2(4):e000037.
64. Fleg JL. Effect of statins alone versus statins plus ezetimibe on carotid atherosclerosis in type 2 diabetes: the SANDS (Stop Atherosclerosis in Native Diabetics Study) trial. J Am Coll Cardiol 2008;52(25):2198–205.
65. Toth PP. Safety profile of statins alone or combined with ezetimibe: a pooled analysis of 27 studies including over 22,000 patients treated for 6-24 weeks. Int J Clin Pract 2012;66(8):800–12.
66. Cannon CP. Rationale and design of IMPROVE-IT (IMProved Reduction of Outcomes: Vytorin Efficacy International Trial): comparison of ezetimbe/simvastatin versus simvastatin monotherapy on cardiovascular outcomes in patients with acute coronary syndromes. Am Heart J 2008;156(5):826–32.
67. Yokoyama M. Effects of eicosapentaenoic acid on major coronary events in hypercholesterolaemic patients (JELIS): a randomised open-label, blinded endpoint analysis. Lancet 2007;369(9567):1090–8.

68. Dietary supplementation with n-3 polyunsaturated fatty acids and vitamin E after myocardial infarction: results of the GISSI-Prevenzione trial. Gruppo Italiano per lo Studio della Sopravvivenza nell'Infarto miocardico. Lancet 1999;354(9177): 447–55.
69. ORIGIN Trial Investigators. n-3 fatty acids and cardiovascular outcomes in patients with dysglycemia. N Engl J Med 2012;367(4):309–18.
70. Risk and Prevention Study Collaborative Group, et al. n-3 fatty acids in patients with multiple cardiovascular risk factors. N Engl J Med 2013;368(19):1800–8.
71. Kromhout D. n-3 fatty acids and cardiovascular events after myocardial infarction. N Engl J Med 2010;363(21):2015–26.
72. Eussen SR. Effects of n-3 fatty acids on major cardiovascular events in statin users and non-users with a history of myocardial infarction. Eur Heart J 2012; 33(13):1582–8.
73. Ballantyne CM. Efficacy and safety of eicosapentaenoic acid ethyl ester (AMR101) therapy in statin-treated patients with persistent high triglycerides (from the ANCHOR study). Am J Cardiol 2012;110(7):984–92.
74. Bays HE. Eicosapentaenoic acid ethyl ester (AMR101) therapy in patients with very high triglyceride levels (from the Multi-center, plAcebo-controlled, Randomized, double-blINd, 12-week study with an open-label Extension [MARINE] trial). Am J Cardiol 2011;108(5):682–90.
75. Kastelein JJ. Omega-3 free fatty acids for the treatment of severe hypertriglyceridemia: the EpanoVa fOr Lowering Very high triglyceridEs (EVOLVE) trial. J Clin Lipidol 2014;8(1):94–106.
76. Maki KC. A highly bioavailable omega-3 free fatty acid formulation improves the cardiovascular risk profile in high-risk, statin-treated patients with residual hypertriglyceridemia (the ESPRIT trial). Clin Ther 2013;35(9):1400–11.e1–3.
77. Rader DJ, Kastelein JJ. Lomitapide and mipomersen: two first-in-class drugs for reducing low-density lipoprotein cholesterol in patients with homozygous familial hypercholesterolemia. Circulation 2014;129(9):1022–32.
78. Blom DJ. A 52-week placebo-controlled trial of evolocumab in hyperlipidemia. N Engl J Med 2014;370(19):1809–19.
79. Raal F. Low-density lipoprotein cholesterol-lowering effects of AMG 145, a monoclonal antibody to proprotein convertase subtilisin/kexin type 9 serine protease in patients with heterozygous familial hypercholesterolemia: the Reduction of LDL-C with PCSK9 Inhibition in Heterozygous Familial Hypercholesterolemia Disorder (RUTHERFORD) randomized trial. Circulation 2012;126(20):2408–17.
80. Roth EM. Atorvastatin with or without an antibody to PCSK9 in primary hypercholesterolemia. N Engl J Med 2012;367(20):1891–900.
81. Stein EA. Effect of a monoclonal antibody to PCSK9, REGN727/SAR236553, to reduce low-density lipoprotein cholesterol in patients with heterozygous familial hypercholesterolaemia on stable statin dose with or without ezetimibe therapy: a phase 2 randomised controlled trial. Lancet 2012;380(9836):29–36.
82. Stroes E. Anti-PCSK9 antibody effectively lowers cholesterol in patients with statin intolerance: the GAUSS-2 randomized, placebo-controlled phase 3 clinical trial of evolocumab. J Am Coll Cardiol 2014;63(23):2541–8.
83. Sullivan D. Effect of a monoclonal antibody to PCSK9 on low-density lipoprotein cholesterol levels in statin-intolerant patients: the GAUSS randomized trial. JAMA 2012;308(23):2497–506.
84. Desai NR. AMG 145, a monoclonal antibody against PCSK9, facilitates achievement of national cholesterol education program-adult treatment panel III low-density lipoprotein cholesterol goals among high-risk patients: an analysis

from the LAPLACE-TIMI 57 trial (LDL-C assessment with PCSK9 monoclonal antibody inhibition combined with statin thErapy-thrombolysis in myocardial infarction 57). J Am Coll Cardiol 2014;63(5):430–3.

85. RUTHERFORD-2: The addition of evolocumab (AMG 145) allows the majority of heterozygous familial hypercholesterolemic patients to achieve low-density lipo-protein cholesterol goals - results from the phase 3 randomized, double-blind, placebo-controlled study. Presented at ACC Scientific Sessions. 2014.

New Therapies for Reducing Low-Density Lipoprotein Cholesterol

Evan A. Stein, MD, PhD[a],*, Frederick J. Raal, MBBCh, MMED, PhD[b]

KEYWORDS

- LDL cholesterol • Apo B antisense • MTP inhibitors • PCSK9 inhibitors

KEY POINTS

- Although the past 4 decades have probably been the most fruitful and productive in transitioning from a low-density lipoprotein (LDL) cholesterol hypothesis to demonstration of clinical benefit, cardiovascular disease still remains the major cause of mortality and morbidity in industrialized societies.
- Cardiovascular disease is rapidly becoming the major cause of morbidity and mortality in recently industrializing countries, like India and China, that together constitute nearly half the world's population.
- It is fortunate that most of the most effective lipid-lowering drugs, the statins, have become, or will soon become, generic and inexpensive.
- There remains a large unmet medical need for new and effective agents that are also well tolerated and safe, especially for patients unable to either tolerate statins or achieve optimal LDL-C on current therapies.

INTRODUCTION

It is now nearly 3 decades since the first HMG CoA reductase inhibitor ("statin") was approved for general use on September 1, 1987, to lower low-density lipoprotein cholesterol (LDL-C).[1] Since that time, the statins have become the cornerstone and mainstay of guidelines in every country to reduce cardiovascular disease.[2–5] Large placebo or comparator trials have clearly demonstrated that statins significantly and substantially reduce morbidity and mortality of all forms of atherosclerotic disease, especially coronary heart disease (CHD) and stroke, no matter what the starting levels of LDL-C and the underlying absolute risk of CHD in the population in the trial.[6] As more effective statins have been developed and approved, with the most effective

[a] Metabolic and Atherosclerosis Research Center, 5355 Medpace Way, Cincinnati, OH 45227, USA; [b] Department of Medicine, Faculty of Health Sciences, University of the Witwatersrand, 7 York Road, Parktown, Johannesburg 2193, South Africa
* Corresponding author.
E-mail address: esteinmrl@aol.com

Endocrinol Metab Clin N Am 43 (2014) 1007–1033
http://dx.doi.org/10.1016/j.ecl.2014.08.008
0889-8529/14/$ – see front matter © 2014 Elsevier Inc. All rights reserved.

of these agents at its highest dose reducing LDL-C by 55% on average, associated CHD outcome trials also have been carried out to show that the lower LDL-C levels attained are associated with lower CHD events.[7,8] The initial statins started becoming available as generic formulations in late 2001, with the major selling agents, simvastatin becoming generic in 2006 and atorvastatin in 2011.[9,10] The last remaining major and most effective statin, rosuvastatin, became generic in a number of countries, such as Canada and Brazil in 2012, and will do so in the United States in 2016 and in Europe a year later.[11] Thus, with generic atorvastatin even at its highest dose now costing less than a cup of coffee a week, even without insurance coverage,[12] and being able to achieve LDL-C reductions on average of 50%, new LDL-C–lowering agents are, and will in the future, be confined to specific situations in which statins are either not tolerated, are contraindicated, or cannot on their own achieve optimal LDL-C reductions.

Patients unable to tolerate statins, effective doses of statins, or achieve optimal control despite statins, currently have limited options that achieve LDL-C–lowering efficacy even in the range of the less effective statins of 2 decades ago. Among the alternative agents are the cholesterol absorption transport inhibitor, ezetimibe, extended release (ER) niacin, bile acid sequestrants, and fibrates. However, these agents reduce LDL-C only by 12% to 18%, may be associated with significant adverse events, and in recent outcome trials have not been shown to further reduce CHD events when added to statins.[13–16]

Therefore, the need for new or additional LDL-C–lowering agents can be summarized as follows (**Box 1**):

1. The largest need is in the large and growing number of statin-adverse patients,[17] in whom there are limited alternatives to achieving significant LDL-C reductions if even low-dose or intermittent-dose statin can be tolerated.[18] During the first 2 decades of statin development and use, the concern for statin toxicity was the severe and life-threatening, although rare, rhabdomyolysis. However, as statin use has grown to tens of millions of the population and extended to primary prevention in high-risk individuals, there has been more attention paid to milder nonspecific myalgias, and other muscle-related side effects (MRSE), as these symptoms are an impediment to maintaining successful long-term lipid-lowering therapy in everyday medical practice. The magnitude of the problem has recently been more fully addressed[19] and estimated to be 5% to 10% of statin-treated patients. With more

---

Box 1
Unmet medical needs for new effective, well-tolerated, and safe low-density lipoprotein-cholesterol (LDL-C)–lowering agents

1. Severe hypercholesterolemia: Despite reduction of 50%–60% with high-dose efficacious stains and ezetimibe, many of the millions of patients with autosomal dominant forms of elevated LDL-C still do not reach optimal levels.

2. Statin intolerance: Although only approximately 5%–10% of patients requiring statins cannot tolerate them, or high enough doses, this constitutes many millions of actual patients.

3. Lower is better: Based on evidence-based clinical trials involving more than 170,000 patients, greater LDL-C reduction results in greater cardiovascular disease (CVD) risk reduction.

4. Treatment guidelines: The overwhelming majority of countries recommend LDL-C treatment goals in patients with high-risk and very high risk CVD, which are often not attainable with current therapies.

than 20 million patients in the United States alone requiring statin therapy or more than a 35% reduction in LDL-C, there are a projected 1 to 2 million patients who will complain of statin side effects and therefore need effective nonstatin LDL-C lowering.

2. There are populations with more severe elevations of LDL-C, such as autosomal dominant hypercholesterolemia (ADH), where most do not achieve optimal levels of LDL-C, despite reductions of 50% to 65% achievable by combining the highest dose of the most effective statins and ezetimibe.[20,21] Recent revisions from 1 in 500 to 1 in 250, based on genetic screening, to the previously thought prevalence of ADH has also further highlighted the unmet need in this population.[22]

3. Pooled analysis by the Cholesterol Treatment Trialists' Collaborators (CTTC) from 27 trials of statin versus placebo or more versus less statin, with 174,149 randomized patients, showed a reduction in the 5-year incidence of major coronary events, coronary revascularizations, and ischemic strokes by approximately 20% for every 40-mg/dL reduction in LDL-C. In addition, greater reductions in LDL-C obtained with more intensive statin regimens further reduced the incidence of major vascular events.[6] Based on this large body of evidence, clinical practice guidelines, with the recent exception of those from the American Heart Association/American College of Cardiology have recommended lower LDL-C goals, currently less than 70 mg/dL, in high-risk patients with CHD.[2–5]

This review describes a number of agents either recently approved or currently in advanced large-scale trials that produce sufficient LDL-C reduction to potentially meet the current unmet needs outlined previously.

LOW-DENSITY LIPOPROTEIN CHOLESTEROL LOWERING AGENTS RECENTLY APPROVED

Although statins increase removal of LDL-C from the circulation, depending to a significant extent on the LDL receptor, an alternative approach is to decrease apolipoprotein (Apo) B containing lipoprotein formation and/or release from the liver and/or the intestines (**Fig. 1**). If inhibition is selective for hepatic Apo B (B_{100}) lipoprotein formation, then very low density lipoprotein (VLDL), intermediate density lipoprotein (IDL), and LDL will be prevented from entering the circulation. If inhibition is nonspecific, then in addition to reduction in B_{100} lipoprotein formation, there will be reductions in Apo B_{48} containing lipoproteins, chylomicrons, and remnants. The 2 current approaches are selective inhibition of hepatic Apo B_{100} synthesis with gene silencing antisense technology and nonselective inhibition of lipidation of Apo B_{100} and B_{48} lipoproteins by the enzyme microsomal triglyceride transport protein (MTP).[23] Mipomersen, an Apo B antisense drug, and lomitapide, an MTP inhibitor, have both recently been approved in the United States by the Food and Drug Administration (FDA) solely for the treatment of homozygous familial hypercholesterolemia (HoFH), although they carry black box warnings about significant side effects (**Table 1**) and are prescribed only under a risk evaluation and mitigation strategy (REMS) program (**Table 2**).[24,25]

Apolipoprotein B Antisense (Mipomersen)

The principle for inhibiting hepatic Apo B_{100} production is shown in **Fig. 2**. Briefly, as for all protein synthesis the process is initiated from deoxyribonucleic acid (DNA), which consists of 2 strands, one representing the "sense" genetic code sequence, and the other strand, containing complementary base pairs, is the "antisense" coding. During transcription, the "sense" and "antisense" strands separate, and the "antisense" strand serves as a template for the next step, which is to produce a single-stranded messenger ribonucleic acid (mRNA). The mRNA also has a base-pairing

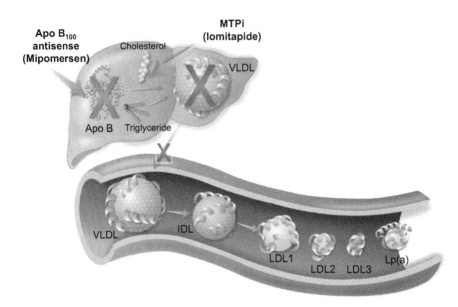

Fig. 1. Inhibition of Apo B100 synthesis and MTP activity. Apo B-100 is an important structural and functional component of lipoproteins. Inhibiting Apo B100 production reduces VLDL, IDL, LDL, and Lp(a) production. MTP is an enzyme required for lipidation of Apo B100 and B48 for formation of VLDL in liver and chylomicrons in gut. Inhibiting MTP reduces hepatic VLDL, IDL, LDL, and intestinal chylomicron formation and remnant production. (*Adapted from* Brautbar A, Ballantyne CM. Pharmacological strategies for lowering LDL cholesterol: statins and beyond. Nat Rev Cardiol 2011;8:253–265; and Parhofer KG. Mipomersen: evidence-based review of its potential in the treatment of homozygous and severe heterozygous familial hypercholesterolemia. Core Evid 2012;7:29–38.)

matching the DNA antisense and is also termed "sense." On reaching the cytosol, ribosomes translate the mRNA to produce proteins, in this case Apo B. By developing agents with RNase activity that will degrade a specific mRNA, it has been possible to impair translation of the downstream protein (see **Fig. 2**). Mipomersen thus binds by Watson and Crick base-pairing and is complementary to a 20-nucleotide segment of the coding region for the mRNA for Apo B. This selective hybridization/binding to its cognate mRNA results in the RNase H-mediated degradation of the Apo B message and inhibits Apo B protein synthesis.[23]

A potential advantage of antisense drugs is their increased specificity for the liver and thus they are best used to inhibit proteins that are predominantly made in the liver, such as Apo B and a number of other proteins important in lipid metabolism, such as Apo CIII, the "small a" component of lipoprotein (a) (Lp(a)), and proprotein convertase subtilisin/kexin type 9 (PCSK9).

All antisense drugs developed to date have been of single-strand antisense nucleotide sequences that are complementary to mRNA, called antisense oligonucleotides or ASOs. The tissue levels are predictable from plasma concentrations, where they are 90% protein bound, and correlate well with the pharmacology of ASOs. They disappear from the bloodstream rapidly but remain in tissue for prolonged periods, often months.

ASOs are generally 20 base-pairs long and behave stably and predictably irrespective of sequence. Mipomersen (ISIS 301012) is the nonadecasodium salt of a 20-base (20-mer) phosphorothioate oligonucleotide. Each of the 19 internucleotide

Table 1
Food and Drug Administration required "boxed warning" for lomitapide and mipomersen regarding risk of hepatotoxicity

Concern	Lomitapide	Mipomersen
Hepatic transaminases	Can cause elevations; 34% of patients in the phase 3 trial had at least one elevation in ALT or AST ≥3 times ULN.	Can cause elevations; 12% of patients in the phase 3 trial treated compared with 0% of the placebo-treated group had at least one elevation in ALT ≥3 times ULN.
Bilirubin, INR, and alkaline phosphatase	No concomitant clinically meaningful elevations.	No concomitant clinically meaningful elevations.
Hepatic fat	Increases hepatic fat, with or without concomitant increases in transaminases. The median absolute increase in hepatic fat was 6% after both 26 and 78 wk of treatment, from 1% at baseline, measured by magnetic resonance spectroscopy.	Increases hepatic fat, with or without concomitant increases in transaminases. In trials with heterozygous FH, the median absolute increase in hepatic fat was 10% after 26 wk of treatment, from 0% at baseline, measured by magnetic resonance imaging.
Hepatic steatosis	Treatment may be a risk factor for progressive liver disease, including steatohepatitis and cirrhosis.	Hepatic steatosis is a risk factor for advanced liver disease, including steatohepatitis and cirrhosis.
Monitoring recommendations	Measure ALT, AST, alkaline phosphatase, and total bilirubin before initiating treatment and then ALT and AST regularly as recommended. During treatment, adjust the dose if the ALT or AST are ≥3 times ULN. Discontinue the drug for clinically significant liver toxicity.	Measure ALT, AST, alkaline phosphatase, and total bilirubin before initiating treatment and then ALT and AST regularly as recommended. During treatment, withhold the dose if the ALT or AST are ≥3 times ULN. Discontinue the drug for clinically significant liver toxicity.

Abbreviations: ALT, alanine aminotransferase; AST, aspartate aminotransferase; FH, familial hyper-cholesterolemia; INR, international normalized ratio; ULN, upper limit of normal.

linkages is a 3′-O to 5′-O phosphorothioate diester. Ten of the 20 sugar residues are 2-deoxy-D-ribose; the remaining 10 are 2-O-(2-methoxyethyl)-D-ribose (MOE). The residues are arranged such that 5 MOE nucleosides at the 5′ and 3′ ends of the molecule flank a gap of ten 2′-deoxynucleosides.[23] Each of the 9 cytosine bases is methylated at the 5-position (MeC). The 2′-methoxyethyl-5-methyluridine (2′-MOE MeU) nucleosides are also designated as 2′-methoxyethylribothymidine (2′-MOE T) and are also termed "second-generation" ASOs. The molecular formula of mipomersen is $C_{230}H_{305}N_{67}O_{122}P_{19}S_{19}Na_{19}$, and the molecular weight is 7594.9 amu.

Mipomersen is the only Apo B antisense drug to have entered clinical development and progressed to approval for any clinical use. Mipomersen is metabolized by nucleases, both endonucleases and exonucleases, and the fragments are excreted in the urine.

Drug-drug interaction is minimal, as there is no CYP 450 metabolism and studies have shown essentially no interaction with statins or ezetimibe.[26] Mipomersen is poorly

Table 2
Risk evaluation and mitigation strategy (REMS) requirements for lomitapide and mipomersen: common features

I. Goals

To educate prescribers about the following:	a. The risk of hepatotoxicity associated with the drugs. b. The need to monitor patients as per product labeling. c. Restricting access to patients with a clinical or laboratory diagnosis consistent with homozygous familial hypercholesterolemia (HoFH).

II. REMS elements

A. Elements to ensure safe use

1. Health care providers (HCPs) who prescribe are specially certified	a. To become specially certified, prescribers must enroll in the drug's REMS program and complete the following:
	  i. Review the prescribing information.
	  ii. Reviewing the materials or module in the REMS Prescriber Education and Enrollment Kit.
	  iii. Complete, sign and submit the prescriber enrollment form.
	b. The drug company will
	  i. Ensure REMS Prescriber Education and Enrollment Kit or Training Module and prescriber enrollment form are on REMS Web site or a coordinating center.
	  ii. Ensure that HCPs complete training and enrollment form before activating prescribers' certification.
	  iii. Inform prescribers of substantive changes to REMS program.
	  iv. Communicate information to HCPs and specific professional associations through their REMS program Web site and *Dear Healthcare Provider* and *Dear Professional Association* letters.

2. The drug will be dispensed only by specially certified pharmacies.	a. The company will ensure that the drug will be dispensed only by certified pharmacies.
	b. To be certified, the pharmacy representative must agree to the following:
	  i. To educate all pharmacy staff involved on the drug's REMS program requirements.
	  ii. Put processes and procedures in place to verify that
	    1. The prescriber is certified in REMS program.
	    2. The drug's REMS prescription authorization form is received for each NEW prescription.
	  iii. To be audited to ensure that all processes and procedures are in place and are being followed for the REMS Program.
	  iv. To provide prescription data to the REMS program.

3. The drug will be dispensed only with evidence or documentation of safe-use conditions.	a. To patients whose prescribers are certified in the REMS Program and *attest* on the REMS prescription authorization form that
	  i. They understand that the drug is indicated as an adjunct to lipid-lowering medications and diet to reduce LDL-C and Apo B in patients with *HoFH*;
	  ii. Affirm that their patient has a clinical or laboratory diagnosis consistent with *HoFH*;
	  iii. They understand that the drug has not, or has not been adequately, studied in patients <18 y of age; and
	  iv. Liver function tests have been obtained as directed in the prescribing information.

(continued on next page)

Table 2 (continued)	

B. Implementation system	a. The companies will ensure that their drug is distributed to and dispensed only by certified pharmacies.
	b. The companies will maintain, monitor, and evaluate the implementation of their REMS program.
	  i. Develop and follow written procedures and scripts to implement the REMS.
	  ii. Maintain a secure, validated database of all certified prescribers and pharmacies that is in compliance with 21 CFR Part 11 regulations.
	  iii. Send confirmation of certification to each certified pharmacy.
	  iv. Maintain a REMS program coordinating center with a call center to support patients, prescribers, and pharmacies.
	  v. Ensure materials listed in their REMS program will be available on a Web site or from a REMS program coordinating center.
	  vi. Update all affected materials and notify enrolled prescribers and certified pharmacies if there are substantive changes to the REMS or REMS program.
	  vii. Monitor and audit the certified pharmacies and institute corrective action if noncompliance is found.

C. Timetable for submission of assessments	Companies will submit REMS assessments to the Food and Drug Administration at 6 mo, 12 mo, and annually thereafter from the date of initial approval.

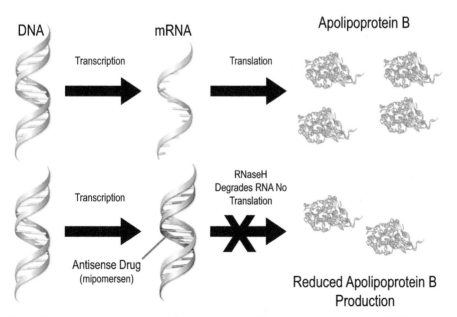

Fig. 2. Mechanism of action: antisense oligonucleotide to reduce hepatic Apo B100 synthesis. (*Adapted from* Goldberg AC. Novel therapies and new targets of treatment for familial hypercholesterolemia. J Clin Lipidol 2010;4(5):353; with permission.)

absorbed from the intestinal tract and is thus administered subcutaneously.[23] Side effects seen in clinical trials appear to be related mostly to the ASOs, and to the mechanism of action: predominantly injection site reactions and liver enzyme elevation.[23]

Mipomersen, and the resultant LDL-C reduction, take up to 6 months to achieve steady state. In early dose-ranging studies[26] carried out in patients with moderately elevated LDL-C on diet alone, mipomersen at dosages of 50, 100, 200, 300, and 400 mg were administered weekly and demonstrated a progressive dose-response-related reduction in LDL-C and Apo B reaching nearly 70% at the 400-mg per week dosage after 12 weeks.[26] Consistent with the long period required to achieve maximal and stable LDL-C reductions, these reductions were sustained even 90 days after cessation of treatment.

Phase 1 and 2 studies performed in patients with heterozygous (He) FH[27] and HoFH[23] in which mipomersen was added to current and maximal lipid therapy showed robust dose-related and time-related reductions in Apo B, triglycerides, non–high-density lipoprotein (HDL)-C and Lp(a) with no significant changes seen in HDL-C or Apo A1. Based on the phase 2 trials, a mipomersen dosage of 200 mg per week was selected for longer and larger phase 3 trials in HeFH[28] and HoFH.[29]

The phase 3 HeFH trial was double-blind, placebo-controlled, and randomized 124 adult patients with coronary artery disease (CAD) on maximally tolerated statin and LDL-C ≥100 mg/dL to mipomersen 200 mg subcutaneously (SC) weekly or placebo (2:1) for 26 weeks. A total of 114 patients, 41/41 on placebo and 73/81 on mipomersen, completed treatment. LDL-C, the primary end point, reduced by a mean (95% confidence interval [CI]) of 28.0% (−34.0% to −22.1%) with mipomersen and increased by 5.2% (−0.5%–10.9%) with placebo, $P<.001$. Mipomersen similarly and significantly reduced Apo B and Apo B containing lipoproteins including Lp(a).[28]

The definitive trial in 51 patients with HoFH, which resulted in the FDA granting marketing approval as an orphan drug for HoFH, was the largest randomized, double-blind, and placebo-controlled trial in this patient population.[29] Seventeen patients were randomized to placebo and 34 to mipomersen 200 mg SC weekly for 26 weeks. Baseline LDL-C concentrations were 400 mg/dL and 439 mg/dL, respectively. Mipomersen treatment resulted in mean (95% CI) LDL-C reductions of 24.7% (−31.6 to −17.7%) compared with a decrease of 3.3% (−12.1%–5.5%) with placebo ($P<.001$), as shown in **Table 3**. Significant ($P<.001$) reductions also were observed

Table 3
Comparative[a] efficacy on LDL-C and other lipoproteins in homozygous FH between microsomal triglyceride transport protein inhibitor (lomitapide), Apo B$_{100}$ antisense inhibitor (mipomersen), and PCSK9 inhibitor (evolocumab)

Parameter	Lomitapide (%)[23,93]	Mipomersen (%)[29]	Evolocumab (%)[80]
LDL-C[b]	−40.1	−21.3	−30.9
Apo B[b]	−39	−24.3	−23.1
Lp(a)[c]	−13.4	−23.2	−11.8
HDL-C[b]	−6.9	+11.2	0
Apo A1[b]	−6.5	+3.9	Not done

Abbreviations: Apo, apolipoprotein; FH, familial hypercholesterolemia; HDL-C, high-density lipoprotein cholesterol; LDL-C, low-density lipoprotein cholesterol; PCSK9, proprotein convertase subtilisin/kexin type 9.
  [a] Based on ITT (intent to treat) analysis and primary/secondary end points from 26-week trials.
  [b] Mean % change (vs placebo for mipomersen and evolocumab, from baseline for lomitapide).
  [c] Median % change.
Data from Refs.[23,29,80,93]

for Apo B (–27%) and Lp(a) (–31%) and HDL-C increased 15% in the mipomersen group (*P* = .035).[29]

Safety and tolerability

The most common adverse events in all trials were injection site reactions, being twice as frequent with mipomersen than placebo in the HeFH trial and 3 times as frequent in patients with HoFH.[28,29] Additional clinically important side effects included flulike symptoms.[23] The most common laboratory findings related to liver function tests: in the HoFH trial, increases of 3 or more times upper limit of normal (ULN) in hepatic transaminases, occurred in 12% of mipomersen-treated patients versus none in the placebo group. In the HeFH trial, hepatic transaminase elevations of 3 or more times ULN occurred in 14.5% mipomersen patients compared with 2.4% on placebo, and in 6.0% of those treated with mipomersen these elevations were confirmed 1 week or more later, whereas none were sustained in placebo patients. One mipomersen-treated patient had maximal alanine aminotransferase of 10 or more times ULN.[28] No patient met Hy's law. A small study had previously demonstrated minimal increases in hepatic triglyceride content as measured by magnetic resonance spectroscopy over 15 weeks of treatment[30]; however, in the phase 3 HeFH trial of 26 weeks, more marked and more frequent hepatitis steatosis was seen with mipomersen.[28] In none of the trials was mipomersen observed to have adverse effects on blood pressure, renal function (serum creatinine, estimated glomerular filtration rate), muscle (myalgia, CK elevation), glucose homeostasis, or platelet count. In the HeFH study, serious adverse events were reported in 4.9% of placebo (CAD and supraventricular tachycardia) and 7.2% of mipomersen-treated patients (basal cell carcinoma, angina pectoris, acute myocardial infarction, chest pain, pulmonary embolism, and noncardiac chest pain). In the HoFH study, serious adverse events were reported in 5.9% in both the placebo and mipomersen groups.

Longer-term and larger studies are needed to determine whether hepatic steatosis will become self-limiting or clinically significant and result in hepatic damage. To address this, "A Study of the Safety and Efficacy of Two Different Regimens of Mipomersen in Patients With Familial Hypercholesterolemia and Inadequately Controlled Low-Density Lipoprotein Cholesterol (FOCUS FH)" commenced in 2011.[31]

Summary

Treatment with mipomersen has been approved only in the United States and is confined to use in HoFH under a strict REMS program (see **Table 2**). The marketing application for HoFH has been submitted in Europe but in December 2012, the Europe Medicines Agency's Committee for Medicinal Products for Human Use (CHMP) rejected the application out of concern that for a drug intended for lifelong use, a high percentage of even homozygous FH patients stopped taking the medicine within 2 years. The CHMP also expressed reservations as to the potential long-term consequences of elevated hepatic transaminases associated with hepatic steatosis and the risk of irreversible liver damage. Along with slightly more cardiovascular events in the mipomersen-treated arms compared with placebo, the agency, at that point in time, felt the benefits of mipomersen did not outweigh its risks and recommended that it be refused marketing authorization.[32] Mipomersen was resubmitted in early 2013 but was again rejected, as the CHMP stated their concerns remained unresolved.[33]

Even though the elevated hepatic transaminases do not appear to reflect drug toxicity and are likely mechanism related from hepatic triglyceride accumulation, this does present a concern for long-term, usually lifelong, therapy. The larger and longer FOCUS FH trial, currently in progress, should provide additional safety information along with information on clinical events.[31] Presumably this will also allow reevaluation by the European agency for homozygous FH. However, even with this information, it is highly unlikely that the use of mipomersen will ever extend to patients without HoFH.

Microsomal Triglyceride Transfer Protein Inhibitors

Microsomal triglyceride transport protein (MTP) is a heterodimeric lipid transfer protein that is localized in the endoplasmic reticulum of hepatocytes and enterocytes and plays a critical role in lipidation of both hepatic Apo B_{100} and intestinal Apo B_{48} (see **Fig. 1**) to form lipoproteins that are then released into the circulation. Without MTP, the formation of chylomicrons, VLDL and their downstream lipoproteins including remnants, IDL, and LDL does not occur.

Inhibition of MTP became a potential therapeutic target following the discovery in 1992 by Wetterau and others[34] of MTP deficiency as the cause of a rare inherited disorder associated with very low levels of LDL-C, called abetalipoproteinemia. Abetalipoproteinemia is also characterized by fat malabsorption, steatorrhea, hepatic steatosis,[35] and neurologic disorders due to the very low levels of Apo B_{48}-containing lipoproteins that transport vitamin E and other lipid-soluble vitamins.[36]

The first MTP inhibitor studied in humans, implitapide (BAY 13-9952), demonstrated significant effects on both hepatic and intestinal lipoproteins within 10 days of exposure.[37] By the early 2000s there were 2 systemic compounds in development: implitapide from Bayer and lomitapide (BMS-201038) from Bristol-Myers Squibb.[38]

Following a large phase 2 trial in Europe with implitapide, the gastrointestinal side effects and hepatic transaminase elevations resulted in Bayer abandoning further development of their compound.[39]

BMS-201038 (lomitapide) was reported in a 7-day multiple ascending-dose, phase-1 study to produce large reductions in LDL-C, ranging from 54% to 86% with doses of 25 to 100 mg per day.[40] A similar effect was seen with implitapide, but a high rate of hepatosteatosis and gastrointestinal adverse experiences were encountered, even with the 25-mg dose in a longer phase 2 trial, the results of which were never published. Subsequently, Bristol-Myers Squibb halted further development.

After being abandoned by major pharmaceutical companies, both implitapide and lomitapide were given to individual academic investigators or academic institutions and small studies to develop them in HoFH and severe HeFH were continued.[40,41] In 2005, lomitapide was licensed by the University of Pennsylvania to Aegerion, and in 2006 the same company obtained implitapide.[42] Lomitapide entered a new phase 2 trial in patients with mildly elevated LDL-C levels at significantly lower starting doses of 5.0 mg daily and after 4 weeks the dose was escalated to 7.5 mg and then to 10.0 mg daily. The reductions in Apo B and LDL-C were dose related and robust. Mean LDL-C decreased 19%, 26%, and 30% at 5.0, 7.5, and 10.0 mg per day respectively (all $P<.01$). As seen for implitapide, statistically significant reductions ranging from 6.5% to 9.2% in HDL-C and 9% to 11% for Apo A1 were reported with all doses over the 12-week trial.[43] The side-effect profile was not favorable, with 32% of patients in the lomitapide monotherapy group discontinuing the trial, mainly for gastrointestinal side effects, which were experienced by 64% of subjects on the drug. Transaminase elevations greater than 3 times ULN occurred in nearly 20% of the patients treated with lomitapide alone or in combination with ezetimibe, resulting in their stopping the drug in the 12-week trial.[43]

Thus, while development of lomitapide was apparently halted for the broad population, a small dose-escalating pilot trial had been done in patients with HoFH.[41] Significant reductions in LDL-C were seen at the higher doses, reaching approximately 50%

at the 55-mg to 80-mg dose. Significant elevations of the hepatic transaminase, alanine aminotransferase, were seen in more than half of the subjects and hepatic magnetic resonance imaging showed hepatic fat accumulation in nearly all patients, with substantial increases seen in some, starting before administration of the highest and most-effective dose.

Following on the results of this proof-of-concept study, and partially funded by the FDA orphan drug program, a larger, open-label phase 3 study of lomitapide in HoFH was undertaken.[44] The study enrolled 29 adult patients, on maximally tolerated lipid-lowering drug therapy, including 16 on LDL apheresis, which remained unchanged during the initial 26 weeks of the trial. Lomitapide was started at a dose of 5 mg per day and titrated at approximately 4-week intervals to a maximum of 60 mg daily. The primary efficacy end point was the LDL-C change at week 26, after which time changes in lipid-lowering therapy were permitted. Six patients terminated with 23 patients completing the 26-week efficacy phase. Based on an intention-to-treat analysis of all 29 patients, the mean LDL-C reduction was 40% from baseline (*P*<.001) with a median dosage of 40 mg per day of lomitapide (see **Table 3**). Individual responses varied even at the same daily dose, similar to the variability seen in HoFH with statins and mipomersen. Parallel reductions in Apo B of 39% and lipoprotein(a) of 13% were seen. Although all the patients were genotyped, the effect of genotype on response was not reported. The result of this open-label trial was the basis for FDA approval in December 2012 of lomitapide solely for the treatment of adults. Similar approval by the European Medicines Agency was obtained in early 2013. The FDA approval carried a black-box warning (see **Table 1**), identical to that for mipomersen, regarding the potential for hepatic toxicity as well as the REMS program, similar to that of mipomersen (see **Table 2**).[24] The FDA also required additional trials in pediatric patients with HoFH, which are ongoing.[24] In addition, as required by the Japanese authorities, a phase 3, open-label trial in Japan of similar design to the trial discussed previously is being performed. This trial is estimated to enroll 5 to 10 adult patients with HoFH receiving concomitant lipid-lowering therapies, including apheresis. Patients will receive lomitapide for 26 weeks, again starting at 5 mg daily and escalating to a maximum dose of 60 mg based on tolerability and hepatic transaminases. Patients will continue into an additional 30-week safety phase with changes in hepatic fat being assessed from baseline to week 56.[45]

Although use of both lomitapide and mipomersen are likely to find a limited role in the treatment of HoFH, it is extremely unlikely, due to their poor tolerability and associated potential for hepatic toxicity, that they will ever become a therapeutic option in less-severe patient populations.

LOW-DENSITY LIPOPROTEIN CHOLESTEROL–LOWERING AGENTS IN ADVANCED CLINICAL DEVELOPMENT

Two therapeutic classes of drugs with LDL-C–lowering potential are currently in phase 3 development. The most exciting are agents inhibiting PCSK9, which, based on supporting genetics, mechanism of action, and larger and predictable reductions in LDL-C, promise to be as revolutionary as the statins were a generation ago, as outlined in detail in the next section.[46] The other class consists of agents that reduce or prevent the exchange of cholesterol between HDL and Apo B containing lipoproteins by inhibiting the enzyme cholesterol ester transfer protein (CETP).[47] The original development concept of CETP inhibitors was to increase HDL-C based on the hypothesis that raising this "anti-atherogenic" lipoprotein would in itself reduce cardiovascular morbidity and mortality. In early trials with the first CETP inhibitor to enter development, torcetrapib, it was noted that LDL-C was concomitantly reduced along with an increase in HDL-C.[48] Minimal, or no reduction in LDL-C was found with a second agent, dalcetrapib, which also raised HDL-C more modestly.[49] These first CETP inhibitors were terminated from clinical development, as outlined later in this article, but 2 additional agents, anacetrapib and evacetrapib, which also produce larger reductions in LDL-C, continue in development.[50,51]

Proprotein Convertase Subtilisin/Kexin Type 9 Inhibitors

In 2003, Abifadel and colleagues[52] described a new form of autosomal dominant hypercholesterolemia (ADH), which was not associated with mutations in the genes coding for the low-density lipoprotein receptor (LDLr) or its ligand, Apo B, but mutations in the gene encoding PCSK9. The role of PCSK9, at that time a recently described member of a nuclear protease family, was unknown and the mechanism by which it impacted LDL-C a complete mystery. By studying transgenic mice that overexpressed PCSK9, Maxwell and Breslow[53] discovered that their LDL receptor (LDLr) function, but not synthesis, was reduced, leading to elevated LDL-C levels. Thus the PCSK9 mutation causing the new form of FH appeared to be due to "gain-of-function" (GOF) in PCSK9, which somehow impacted LDLr function but not production. Additional GOF mutations in PCSK9 leading to elevated LDL-C have since been identified (**Fig. 3**). However, how PCSK9 decreased LDLr activity was not clear, but it did not appear to be due to reduced receptor synthesis, as LDLr mRNA production was unchanged.[54] These observations were soon followed by studies by Rashid and colleagues,[55] in which PCSK9 production was eliminated using a knockout mouse model and LDLr activity was substantially increased with resultant LDL-C reduction. Further studies in humans by Cohen and colleagues[56] confirmed that participants in a large longitudinal epidemiologic cardiovascular study with low plasma levels of LDL-C had "loss-of-function" (LOF) mutations in PCSK9. These families were reported to have a significant reduction in lifetime risk of coronary heart disease, and no adverse health effects. A number of LOF mutations have now been described associated with both reduced LDL-C and risk of cardiovascular disease (CVD) (see **Fig. 3**, **Table 4**). These observations of no adverse health

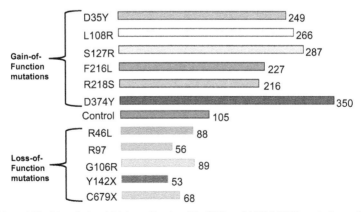

Fig. 3. Mean LDL-C levels (mg/dL) in patients with GOF and LOF PCSK9 mutations. (*Adapted from* Poirier S, Mayer G. The biology of PCSK9 from the endoplasmic reticulum to lysosomes: new and emerging therapeutics to control low-density lipoprotein cholesterol. Drug Des Devel Ther 2013;7:1136.)

Table 4
Risk of early myocardial infarction in subjects with PCSK9 loss-of-function, missense mutation R46L in different populations

Country	Study	Odds Ratio (95% CI)	P Value
Finland	FINRISK	0.30 (0.11–0.81)	.02
Sweden	Malmo: Cardiovascular cohort	0.32 (0.07–1.61)	.17
Spain	REGICOR	0.35 (0.15–0.82)	.02
USA (Seattle)	Puget Sound: heart attack risk	0.45 (0.21–0.98)	.049
USA (Boston)	Massachusetts General: study premature CAD	0.59 (0.21–1.69)	.46
Combined		0.40 (0.26–0.61)	.00002

Abbreviations: CI, confidence interval; PCSK9, proprotein convertase subtilisin/kexin type 9.

Adapted from Kathiresan S, the Myocardial Infarction Genetics Consortium. A PCSK9 missense variant associated with a reduced risk of early-onset myocardial infarction. N Engl J Med 2008;358:2299; with permission.

effects with LOF have been further supported by reports in now a number of healthy unrelated subjects with homozygous or compound heterozygous LOF mutations in PCSK9 and extremely low LDL-C levels, lower than 20 mg/dL, and undetectable PCSK9, essentially equivalent to the mouse PCSK9 model.[57] The mechanism by which PCSK9 reduced LDLr activity was elucidated by Lagace and coworkers in 2006,[58] when they demonstrated that circulating or plasma PCSK9 bound to the LDLr was internalized along with the receptor and LDL-C and targeted the LDLr for degradation (**Fig. 4**), thus preventing the LDLr from recycling back to the cell surface. This provided the critical information needed to design possible methods to inhibit PCSK9 and rapidly lead to development of a monoclonal antibody (mAb) targeted to PCSK9 knowing that preventing PCSK9 in the plasma from binding to the LDLr could restore or increase LDLr activity (see **Fig. 4**C). Proof-of-concept studies in mice and nonhuman primates showed the approach to be effective in binding PCSK9 and reducing LDL-C.[59] As total and free PCSK9 plasma levels can be measured and monitored in plasma it also provided a unique ability to monitor the effect of mAb on both the "target" and LDL-C. Over the past decade, much has been learned about the production and metabolism of PCSK9 before it enters the circulation. PCSK9 is produced mainly by hepatocytes as proPCSK9 in the endoplasmic reticulum and synthesis appears to be mediated via the same transcription factor, sterol receptor element binding protein-2 (SREBP2), which leads to increased synthesis of the LDLr. As plasma PCSK9 ultimately results in degradation of LDLr, this action is mostly likely a counter-regulatory mechanism designed to prevent excessive uptake of cholesterol into liver cells, as the adrenal and other organs in need of LDL-C delivery do not appear to be affected by PCSK9. However, as SREBP2 is upregulated by inhibition of intracellular cholesterol synthesis, for example by HMG CoA reductase inhibitors or "statins," leading to simultaneous increased production of LDLr and PCSK9, it has been postulated that the log linear dose response seen with statins may be due, at least in part, to concomitant reduction in LDLr recycling.[60] In 2009, 2 fully human mAbs, alirocumab and evolocumab, targeted to PCSK9, were being tested in humans.[61,62] The results of the single and multiple ascending dose, phase 1, trials were published in early 2012 demonstrating that administration of a PCSK9 mAb led to dramatic reductions in LDL-C in a broad range of patient phenotypes, whether added to diet alone or to background statin therapy.[61,62] Over the past 2 years, clinical development has progressed very rapidly with 3 mAbs already

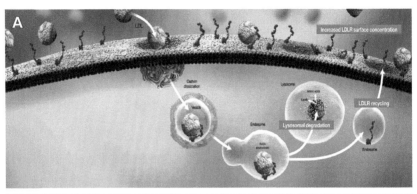

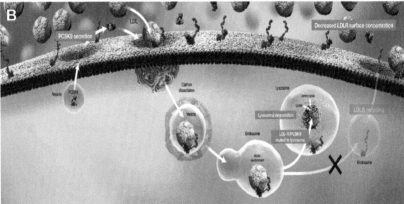

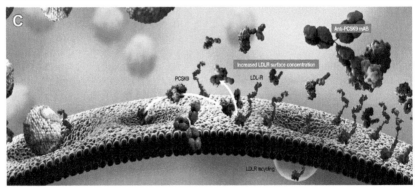

Fig. 4. LDLr, PCSK9, and mAbs to PCSK9 role in receptor function and recycling. (*A*) Normal LDLr recycling. (*B*) Effect of PCSK9 on LDLr recycling. (*C*) Impact of monoclonal antibody to PCSK9 on LDLr recycling. (*From* Stein EA, Wasserman SM, Dias C, et al. AMG-145. Drugs Future 2013;38:453; with permission.)

in phase 3 clinical development.[63–65] The most advanced of these are Amgen's evolocumab (AMG 145) followed by alirocumab (REGN 727/SAR 236553), originally produced by Regeneron and being codeveloped with Sanofi. Comprehensive data have been published on the phase 1 and 2 trials of both drugs,[61,62,66–72] as well as a number of trials from the evolocumab phase 3 program.[73–76] The phase 1b, multiple ascending dose (MAD) program of alirocumab incorporated a number of novel elements that accelerated the knowledge and future clinical development by including patients on stable statin therapy, which is known to increase plasma PCSK9, subjects on diet alone, and patients with HeFH and non-FH.[61] Three different doses, 50, 100, and 150 mg, were administered subcutaneously at differing intervals of 2 and 4 weeks. Using standardized "biomarker" measurements allowed a unique opportunity for direct measurement during these early trials, making it possible to assess the pharmacokinetics and pharmacodynamics by monitoring the mAb, the level of free/unbound PCSK9, and the biomarker of clinical importance, namely LDL-C (**Fig. 5**), in the bloodstream. Even in this fairly small phase 1 trial, it was clear that there was no difference in LDL-C reduction between patients with FH and non-FH, or between those on background statin therapy and those on modified diet alone. By pooling the different patient phenotypes it was also feasible to assess dose response and dose scheduling (ie, dosing at 2-week or 4-week intervals). Although there was a large difference in LDL-C reduction between the 50-mg and 100-mg doses, there was virtually no difference in maximal LDL-C reduction between the 100-mg and 150-mg doses.[61] This indicated, and subsequent studies later confirmed, that nearly all the plasma PCSK9 was bound by the mAb at the 100-mg dose. The effect on LDL-C was rapid, reaching maximum effect within approximately 5 to 7 days after the dose and the reduced LDL-C levels were stable for approximately 2 weeks before free PCSK9 levels started increasing followed quickly by LDL-C. It was also apparent from this limited study that the higher the dose of mAb, the longer the duration of effect, consistent with excess mAb not initially bound to PCSK9 remaining available to bind newly synthesized PCSK9, preventing PCSK9 binding to the LDLr and maintaining lower LDL-C. A similar MAD study with the Amgen monoclonal antibody to PCSK9, evolocumab (AMG 145), in terms of patient phenotypes and background treatments, but with higher doses, and dosing intervals ranging from 1 to 4 weeks, produced almost identical results.[62] Both drugs were well tolerated and had no significant or unexpected clinical or laboratory side effects, and the drugs moved rapidly into larger phase 2 trials in 2011. The results of 3 alirocumab and 4 evolocumab phase 2 trials were published in 2012. The trials can be best summarized by the questions they answered. McKenney and colleagues[66] highlighted 2 issues, whether even higher doses than tested in phase 1 would result in greater LDL-C reduction, prolonged duration of reduction, or both. The study assessed the

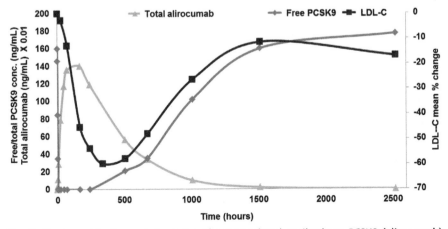

Fig. 5. Pharmacokinetics and dynamics of a monoclonal antibody to PCSK9 (alirocumab), free PCSK9, and LDL-C.

same 100-mg and 150-mg alirocumab doses administered every 2 weeks and compared them with 200 and 300 mg given every 4 weeks. It clearly demonstrated that despite the very large increase of mAb administered, there was no further reduction in LDL-C at any time after dosing. Although the duration of effect with the higher doses of even 300 mg was still not sufficient to maintain for 4 weeks the reductions in LDL-C seen at 2 weeks, there still remained the potential that even larger doses, if practical and cost-effective, could provide a long enough duration of effect to merit 4-week dosing. This was in fact assessed with evolocumab in 2 large studies that used doses up to 420 mg administered every 4 weeks and compared them with lower doses given every 2 weeks.[68,69] As shown in **Fig. 6**, from a pooled and very robust analysis of these trials, when evolocumab was given at a dosage of 420 mg every 4 weeks, the approximate 60% reductions in LDL-C were sustained, with minimal increase between weeks 2 and 4.[77] These data indicated that with high enough dosing there is potential to achieve excellent reductions with monthly therapy with a rough 3-to-1 "rule of thumb" in that 420 mg every 4 weeks would achieve the same stable LDL-C reductions as 140 mg every 2 weeks.

To assess (1) if the "rule of 6s," dose response with statins was due to upregulation of PCSK9 and (2) if there was a maximum to which LDLr activity could be upregulated with statin/PCSK9 mAb combination, Roth and colleagues[67] compared patients on stable doses of atorvastatin 10 mg daily, who were randomized to receive 80 mg of atorvastatin plus alirocumab or placebo or to remain on atorvastatin 10 mg plus alirocumab. The eightfold increase of atorvastatin from 10 to 80 mg alone followed the "rule of 6s" and resulted in the anticipated roughly 18% further reduction in LDL-C. The addition of 150 mg of alirocumab every 2 weeks to the group that maintained atorvastatin 10 mg daily resulted in a 66% decrease in LDL-C from baseline, or a 49% difference from the 80-mg dose of atorvastatin. The group that increased atorvastatin to 80 mg combined with the 150 mg of alirocumab experienced a decrease in LDL-C of 73%, a 55% additional decrease compared with atorvastatin 80 mg alone. The net reduction between 10 and 80 mg atorvastatin combined with the same dose of alirocumab was therefore only 6%.[67] Thus, although inhibiting PCSK9 in patients on maximal-dose atorvastatin was still very effective, the effect was definitely not synergistic, and not even additive, and ruled out the role of PCSK9 as the reason for the log-linear dose response seen with statin dosing. The trial also suggested that there may well be a point at which further upregulation of the LDLr is not possible.

Two trials in HeFH patients, 1 with alirocumab and 1 with evolocumab, assessed if the response seen in the small phase 1 trials in HeFH would be consistent in a global population with FH and more diverse LDLr defects.[68,71] In both trials, the mAb was added to stable treatment of high-dose effective statins and ezetimibe. The trials differed in that the alirocumab study used lower dose, 100 and 150 mg, dosed at 2 weeks, and 200 and 300 mg at 4-week intervals, whereas the evolocumab trial assessed 2 larger doses, 350 mg and 420 mg, given every 4 weeks. Both trials showed excellent mean LDL-C reductions of 60% to 70%, with responses fairly uniform in all FH patients.[68,71]

The final question to be assessed in the phase 2 program was to determine if patients unable to tolerate statins or high doses of statins would tolerate a PCSK9 mAb. The trial of evolocumab used ezetimibe as a nonstatin control group, and enrolled patients with documented muscle-related side effects on at least 1 statin.[72] The study also confirmed the need for additional effective lipid-lowering agents, as baseline LDL-C was close to 200 mg/dL with most patients having CHD or at high risk. The reductions in LDL-C seen across the various doses of evolocumab were consistent with those seen in previous populations, with reductions approaching

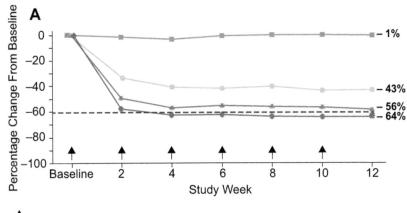

Administration of investigational product

■ Placebo (n = 123)   ▲ AMG 145 105 mg (n = 125)
● AMG 145 70 mg (n = 124) ◆ AMG 145 140 mg (n = 123)

Mean percentage change from baseline in calculated LDL-C.

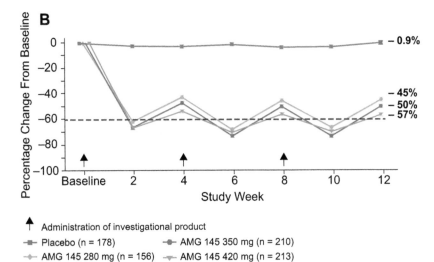

Administration of investigational product

■ Placebo (n = 178)   ● AMG 145 350 mg (n = 210)
◆ AMG 145 280 mg (n = 156) ▼ AMG 145 420 mg (n = 213)

Mean percentage change from baseline in calculated LDL-C.

Fig. 6. (*A*) Evolocumab (AMG 145) every 2 weeks: LDL-C percentage change from baseline. (*B*) Evolocumab (AMG 145) every 4 weeks: LDL-C percentage change from baseline. (*From* Stein EA, Giugliano RP, Koren MJ, et al. Efficacy and safety of evolocumab (AMG 145), a fully human monoclonal antibody to PCSK9, in hyperlipidaemic patients on various background lipid therapies: pooled analysis of 1359 patients in 4 phase 2 trials. Eur Heart J 2014;35:2253; with permission.)

55% with evolocumab 420 mg every 4 weeks. Few patients stopped the study, evolocumab was well tolerated, and minimal elevations in the muscle enzyme creatine kinase were seen.[72]

Reductions in LDL-C have been accompanied by parallel large reductions in Apo B, although the decrease in Apo B is approximately 6% lower than that for LDL-C at any given dose, similar to what is seen with statins.[77] A novel and unexpected finding, consistent in all trials, is an as-yet-unexplained reduction in Lp(a), in the 25% to 30% range (**Fig. 7**).[78]

Consistent with upregulation of LDLr and removal of Apo B–containing lipoproteins, including triglyceride-rich, small, very-low-density and intermediate-density lipoproteins, has been the finding of modest reductions in triglycerides. As anticipated, with improved clearance of LDL-C there have been modest increases in HDL-C and its major constituent apolipoprotein A1.[77]

The last question addressed in phase 2 was to determine if patients with HoFH would respond to PCSK9 inhibition. This was assessed in a small open-label pilot trial of 8 patients: 6 LDLr defective status and 2 with negative LDLr function.[79] Somewhat counter to expectations, a moderate approximate 20% reduction in LDL-C was seen with the response confined to those patients with some residual LDLr activity. The study achieved sufficient response to warrant a large definitive phase 3 trial in patients with HoFH.[80]

More than 1600 patients were randomized between the Sanofi/Regeneron and Amgen programs, with more than 1200 patients treated with active drug, most for 12 weeks. To view this in the context of statin development, the phase 2 trials were

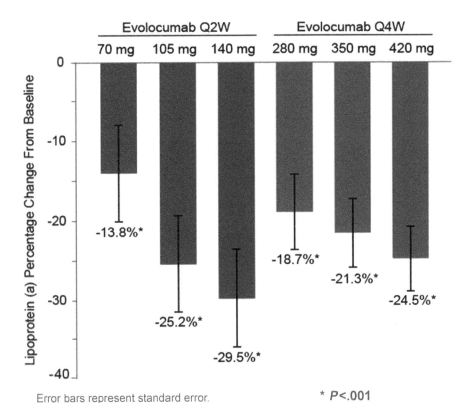

Fig. 7. Reduction in lipoprotein (a) with PCSK9 monoclonal antibody evolocumab (AMG 145): a pooled analysis of more than 1300 patients in 4 phase II trials. (*From* Raal FJ, Giugliano RP, Sabatine MS, et al. Reduction in lipoprotein (a) with the PCSK9 monoclonal antibody evolocumab (AMG 145): a pooled analysis of over 1300 patients in 4 phase 2 trials. J Am Coll Cardiol 2014;63(13):1284; with permission.)

generally 4 or 6 weeks long and fairly small, usually fewer than 100 patients. Thus, by the end of the phase 2 PCSK9 program for these 2 agents, the patient exposure likely exceeds that of all statins combined at the same stage of development. Even though the drugs are administered by SC injection, tolerability has been good, and patients terminating trials no higher than that of statin or other oral lipid-lowering drugs. Elevations of liver function and muscle enzymes seen with statins and some other lipid-lowering drugs have been minimal with PCSK9 mAbs.[77] Nonspecific adverse effects have been reported, although the frequency in the trials has not been noticeably different from placebo or control therapy. Both alirocumab and evolocumab monoclonal antibodies are fully humanized, which minimizes the potential for immune reactions and the development of consistent or high titers of neutralizing antibodies to the agents has not been seen in phase 2 trials.

Concern has been raised regarding very low levels of LDL-C that are achieved in some patients. Although it is reassuring from the epidemiologic studies and the few patients with genetic abnormalities leading to lifelong very low LDL-C, this question will be answered only by the long-term clinical outcome trials currently ongoing in phase 3.[63–65] Alirocumab and evolocumab are now well into large phase 3 programs, with 6 evolocumab trials already published or publically presented.[73–76,78] The major purpose of phase 3 is to assess long-term safety in a larger population so as to provide sufficient information for regulatory agencies to determine the risk to benefit in approving an LDL-C–lowering agent for general use. Thus, little additional information is anticipated with regard to efficacy, which is solidly established and robust in terms of LDL-C reduction and in itself an approvable end point, as recently reiterated by the FDA. However, unlike the long hiatus between development and marketing approval of statins where CHD and clinical outcome trials were only started many years after release general use, evolocumab, alirocumab, and the Pfizer humanized PCSK9 mAb, bococizumab, have already entered large CVD outcome trials as part of their phase 3 programs (**Table 5**).[63–65,81] The first of these trials is anticipated to conclude in late 2016 or early 2017.

To summarize the highlights from the phase 3 trials of evolocumab results available to date, the following can be stated. (1) LDL-C efficacy after 52 weeks was consistent with that seen in the 12-week phase 2.[73] (2) LDL-C efficacy was consistent across a wide spectrum of background therapies including diet alone, various statin doses, to statin plus ezetimibe.[73,76] (3) Trials comparing 140 mg every 2 weeks to 420 mg monthly with assessments at both 2 and 4 weeks after dosing confirmed equivalent LDL-C reductions consistent with the "rule of 3" regarding the 2-week dose needed to achieve stability for 4 weeks.[74,76] (4) Patients intolerant to at least 2 statins still tolerated evolocumab and had the same 60% reductions in LDL-C seen in the phase 2 statin intolerant trial.[75] (5) the definitive double-blind randomized trial in HoFH involving 49 patients showed an overall 31% mean reduction in LDL-C with evolocumab compared with placebo (see **Table 3**), and 40% in those patients with at least 1 LDLr defective allele.[81] (6) Perhaps most important, tolerability and safety continues to be good with no additional findings from the phase 2 studies.

In summary, PCSK9 mAb therapy appears to be the most promising therapeutic class since statins and is able to fill the current medical need outlined in the introduction. Despite the mode of administration by SC injection, and the likely high cost associated with biological agents, the substantial reduction in LDL-C and self-administration of these drugs either every 2 or 4 weeks will likely result in PCSK9 mAbs being widely accepted and used by patients. It is anticipated that the addition of PCSK9 mAbs to current therapy in the CHD outcome trials currently in progress will augment the reductions in CVD that have been achieved by statins.

Table 5
PCSK9 monoclonal antibody cardiovascular outcome trials currently in progress

	Evolocumab (AMG 145)	Alirocumab (SAR236553/REGN727)	Bococizumab (RN 316)	
Sponsor	Amgen	Sanofi/Regeneron	Pfizer	
Trial	FOURIER	ODYSSEY Outcomes	SPIRE I	SPIRE II
Sample size	22,500	18,000	12,000	6300
Patients	MI, stroke, or PAD	4–52 wk post-ACS	High risk of CV event	
Statin	Atorva ≥20 mg or equiv	Evidence-based medicine Rx	Lipid-lowering Rx	
LDL-C mg/dL (mmol/L)	≥70 (≥1.8)	≥70 (≥1.8)	70–99 (1.8–2.6)	≥100 (≥2.6)
PCSK9i Dosing	Q2W or Q4W	Q2W	Q2W	
End point	1. CV death, MI, stroke, revasc or hosp for UA 2. CV death, MI, or stroke	CHD death, MI, ischemic stroke, or hosp for UA	CV death, MI, stroke, or urgent revasc	
Completion	12/2017	1/2018	8/2017	

Abbreviations: ACS, acute coronary syndrome; CHD, coronary heart disease; CV, cardiovascular; hosp, hospitalization; MI, myocardial infarction; PAD, peripheral arterial disease; PCSK9, propro-tein convertase subtilisin/kexin type 9; revasc, revascularization; Rx, prescription; UA, unstable angina.

An alternative therapeutic approach to mAbs using the similar antisense technology described previously for Apo B was demonstrated in an animal model,[82] in which a second-generation antisense ASO directed at murine PCKS9 reduced PCSK9 expression and decreased LDLc by 38% in 6 weeks. Despite the promise shown in these animal experiments, combined with the human experience with the Apo B ASO, mipomersen, and a partnership announced in 2007 between ISIS Pharmaceuticals and Bristol-Myers Squibb,[83] this approach has not entered human trials. An alternative method for gene "silencing" by using short interfering RNA has been developed by Alnylam. In a proof-of-concept single ascending dose study, both plasma PCSK9 and LDL-C reductions were reported.[84]

Cholesterol Ester Transfer Protein Inhibitors

CETP, a plasma protein that catalyzes the exchange of cholesteryl esters and triglyceride between HDL and Apo B containing lipoproteins, was identified as a potential therapeutic target from populations with elevated HDL-C and apparent reduction in CVD risk.[85] Subsequently, genetic mutations in CETP were found to be related to elevations in HDL-C and pharmacologic inhibition was able to reproduce a similar elevation.[48,85] Along with the increase in HDL-C, it was noted that there was a reduction in LDL-C, which mechanistically was consistent with the prevention of cholesterol transfer from HDL to LDL.[48] The magnitude of LDL-C reduction has varied with different CETP inhibitors, as well as with the dose of specific inhibitors.[86,87] For example, minimal or no LDL-C reduction was seen with dalcetrapib, to moderate reductions of approximately 20% with torcetrapib.[48,49] Both of these agents were terminated after large CVD outcome trials were stopped, for toxicity in the case of torcetrapib and futility in the case of dalcetrapib.[50,51] However 2 CETP inhibitors, evacetrapib and anacetrapib, continue in development, both now in large CVD outcome trials.[88,89]

Anacetrapib, a potent and selective CETP inhibitor at 150 and 300 mg daily, increased HDL-C and Apo A-I of 39% and 47%, respectively. At dosages of 10, 40, 150, and 300 mg daily, LDL-C reductions ranged from 15% to approximately 40%.[90] A dose of 100 mg was selected for the CVD outcome trial, which in a large trial lowered LDL-C by 25% to 35%.[91,92] This dose is also being used in the large 30,624-patient CVD outcome trial, REVEAL (Randomized EValuation of the Effects of Anacetrapib Through Lipid-modification), currently in progress with results anticipated in 2017.[89]

Evacetrapib, also a potent inhibitor of CETP, showed a dose response in both HDL-C and LDL-C in a dose ranging trial with increases of HDL-C of 54%, 95%, and 129%, and reductions in LDL-C of 14%, 22%, and 36% with doses of 30, 100, and 500 mg per day.[87] A dose of 130 mg was selected for the 12,000-patient ACCELERATE CVD outcome trial currently in progress, with results expected in late 2016.[88]

Depending on the results, it may be that these agents would be used to reduce LDL-C, although their primary action is to increase HDL-C and their effect on LDL-C is relatively small compared with PCSK9 inhibitors.

SUMMARY

Although the past 4 decades have probably been the most fruitful and productive in transitioning from an LDL-C hypothesis to demonstration of clinical benefit, CVD still remains the major cause of mortality and morbidity in industrialized societies. It is rapidly becoming the major cause of morbidity and mortality in recently industrializing countries, such as India and China, that together constitute nearly half of the world's population. It is fortunate that most of the most-effective lipid-lowering drugs, the statins, have become, or will soon become, generic and very inexpensive. However, there remains a large unmet medical need for new and effective agents that are also well tolerated and safe, especially for patients unable to either tolerate statins or achieve optimal LDL-C on current therapies. It is likely that the agents discussed in this review will fill that need.

REFERENCES

1. Statins: a success story involving FDA, academia and industry. Available at: http://www.fda.gov/AboutFDA/WhatWeDo/History/ProductRegulation/Selections FromFDLIUpdateSeriesonFDAHistory/ucm082054.htm. Accessed July 25, 2014.
2. Stone N, Robinson J, Lichtenstein AH, et al. 2013 ACC/AHA guideline on the treatment of blood cholesterol to reduce atherosclerotic cardiovascular risk in adults: a report of the American College of Cardiology/American Heart Association Task Force on Practice Guidelines. Circulation 2014;129:S1–45.
3. European Association for Cardiovascular Prevention & Rehabilitation, Reiner Z, Catapano AL, et al, ESC Committee for Practice Guidelines (CPG) 2008-2010 and 2010-2012 Committees. ESC/EAS Guidelines for the management of dyslipidaemias: the Task Force for the management of dyslipidaemias of the European Society of Cardiology (ESC) and the European Atherosclerosis Society (EAS). Eur Heart J 2011;32:1769–818.
4. Anderson TJ, Grégoire J, Hegele RA, et al. 2012 Update of the Canadian Cardiovascular Society guidelines for the diagnosis and treatment of dyslipidemia for the prevention of cardiovascular disease in the adult. Can J Cardiol 2013; 29:151–67.

5. National Heart Foundation of Australia and the Cardiac Society of Australia and New Zealand. Reducing risk in heart disease: an expert guide to clinical practice for secondary prevention of coronary heart disease. Melbourne (Australia): National Heart Foundation of Australia; 2012. Available at: http://www.heartfoundation.org.au/SiteCollectionDocuments/Reducing-risk-inheart-disease.pdf. Accessed July 10, 2014.

6. Cholesterol Treatment Trialists' (CTT) Collaboration, Baigent C, Blackwell L, et al. Efficacy and safety of more intensive lowering of LDL cholesterol: a meta-analysis of data from 170,000 participants in 26 randomised trials. Lancet 2010;376:1670–81.

7. Jones PH, Davidson MH, Stein EA, et al, STELLAR Study Group. Comparison of efficacy and safety of rosuvastatin versus atorvastatin, simvastatin, and pravastatin across doses (STELLAR Trial). Am J Cardiol 2003;92:152–60.

8. LaRosa JC, Grundy SM, Waters DD, et al, Treating to New Targets (TNT) Investigators. Intensive lipid lowering with atorvastatin in patients with stable coronary disease. N Engl J Med 2005;352(14):1425–35.

9. Billups SJ, Plushner SL, Olson KL, et al. Clinical and economic outcomes of conversion of simvastatin to lovastatin in a group-model health maintenance organization. J Manag Care Pharm 2005;11(8):681–6.

10. Jackevicius CA, Chou MM, Ross JS, et al. Generic atorvastatin and health care costs. N Engl J Med 2012;366(3):201–4.

11. Howard L. Drug in focus: rosuvastatin. Available at: http://www.genericsweb.com/index.php?object_id=680. Accessed July 12, 2014.

12. Available at: http://www2.costco.com/Pharmacy/DrugInfo.aspx?p=1&SearchTerm=atorvastatin&Drug=ATORVASTATIN. Accessed July 12, 2014.

13. Ezzet F, Wexler D, Statkevich P, et al. The plasma concentration and LDL-C relationship in patients receiving ezetimibe. J Clin Pharmacol 2001;41(9):943–9.

14. Davidson MH, Dillon MA, Gordon B, et al. Colesevelam hydrochloride (cholestagel): a new, potent bile acid sequestrant associated with a low incidence of gastrointestinal side effects. Arch Intern Med 1999;159(16):1893–900.

15. Capuzzi DM, Guyton JR, Morgan JM, et al. Efficacy and safety of an extended-release niacin (Niaspan): a long-term study. Am J Cardiol 1998;82(12A):74U–81U.

16. Knopp RH, Brown WV, Dujovne CA, et al. Effects of fenofibrate on plasma lipoproteins in hypercholesterolemia and combined hyperlipidemia. Am J Med 1987;83(5B):50–9.

17. Maningat P, Gordon BR, Breslow JL. How do we improve patient compliance and adherence to long-term statin therapy? Curr Atheroscler Rep 2013;15(1):291.

18. Stein EA, Ballantyne CM, Windler E, et al. Efficacy and tolerability of Fluvastatin XL 80 mg alone, ezetimibe alone and the combination of Fluvastatin XL 80 mg with ezetimibe in patients with a history of muscle-related side effects with other statins: a randomized, double-blind, double-dummy trial. Am J Cardiol 2008;101:490–6.

19. Bruckert E, Hayem G, Dejager S, et al. Mild to moderate muscular symptoms with high-dosage statin therapy in hyperlipidemic patients—the PRIMO study. Cardiovasc Drugs Ther 2005;19:403–14.

20. Stein E, Stender S, Mata P, et al, Ezetimibe Study Group. Achieving lipoprotein goals in patients at high risk with severe hypercholesterolemia: efficacy and safety of ezetimibe co-administered with atorvastatin. Am Heart J 2004;148(3):447–55.

21. Stein EA, Ose L, Retterstol K, et al. Further reductions in low-density lipoprotein cholesterol and C-reactive protein with the addition of ezetimibe to maximum dose rosuvastatin in patients with severe hypercholesterolemia. J Clin Lipidol 2007;1:280–6.

22. Nordestgaard BG, Chapman MJ, Humphries SE, et al. Familial hypercholesterolaemia is underdiagnosed and undertreated in the general population: guidance for clinicians to prevent coronary heart disease. Eur Heart J 2013;34:3478–90.

23. Rader DJ, Kastelein JJ. Lomitapide and mipomersen: two first-in-class drugs for reducing low-density lipoprotein cholesterol in patients with homozygous familial hypercholesterolemia. Circulation 2014;129:1022–32.

24. FDA approves new orphan drug for rare cholesterol disorder. US Food and Drug Administration Web site. 2012. Available at: http://www.fda.gov/NewsEvents/ Newsroom/PressAnnouncements/ucm333285.htm. Accessed May 28, 2014.

25. FDA approves new orphan drug Kynamro to treat inherited cholesterol disorder. US Food and Drug Administration Web site. 2013. Available at: http://www.fda. gov/NewsEvents/Newsroom/PressAnnouncements/ucm337195.htm. Accessed May 28, 2014.

26. Kastelein JJ, Wedel MK, Baker BF, et al. Potent reduction of apolipoprotein B and low-density lipoprotein cholesterol by short-term administration of an antisense inhibitor of apolipoprotein B. Circulation 2006;114:1729–35.

27. Akdim F, Visser ME, Tribble DL, et al. Effect of mipomersen, an apolipoprotein B synthesis inhibitor, on low-density lipoprotein cholesterol in patients with familial hypercholesterolemia. Am J Cardiol 2010;105:1413–9.

28. Stein EA, Dufour R, Gagne C, et al. Apolipoprotein B synthesis inhibition with mipomersen in heterozygous familial hypercholesterolemia: results of a randomized, double-blind, placebo-controlled trial to assess efficacy and safety as add-on therapy in patients with coronary artery disease. Circulation 2012;126:2283–92.

29. Raal FJ, Santos RD, Blom DJ, et al. Mipomersen, an apolipoprotein B synthesis inhibitor, for lowering of LDL cholesterol concentrations in patients with homozygous familial hypercholesterolaemia: a randomised, double-blind, placebo-controlled trial. Lancet 2010;375:998–1006.

30. Visser ME, Akdim F, Tribble DL, et al. Effect of apolipoprotein-B synthesis inhibition on liver triglyceride content in patients with familial hypercholesterolemia. J Lipid Res 2010;51(5):1057–62.

31. A Study of the safety and efficacy of two different regimens of mipomersen in patients with familial hypercholesterolemia and inadequately controlled low-density lipoprotein cholesterol (FOCUS FH). Available at: http://clinicaltrials. gov/show/NCT01475825. Accessed July 12, 2014.

32. Available at: http://www.ema.europa.eu/docs/en_GB/document_library/Summary_ of_opinion_-_Initial_authorisation/human/002429/WC500140678.pdf.   Accessed July 12, 2014.

33. Available   at: http://www.forbes.com/sites/larryhusten/2013/03/22/europe-and-us-diverge-on-two-new-drugs/. Accessed July 12, 2014.

34. Wetterau JR, Aggerbeck LP, Bouma ME, et al. Absence of microsomal triglyceride transfer protein in individuals with abetalipoproteinemia. Science 1992;258: 999–1001.

35. Scriver CR, Sly WS, Childs B, et al, editors. The metabolic and molecular bases of inherited disease. 8th edition. McGraw-Hill Professional; 2000.

36. Rader DJ, Brewer HB Jr. Abetalipoproteinemia: new insights into lipoprotein assembly and vitamin E metabolism from a rare genetic disease. JAMA 1993;270: 865–9.

37. Stein EA, Isaacsohn JL, Mazzu A, et al. Effect of BAY 13-9952, a microsomal tri-glyceride transfer protein inhibitor on lipids and lipoproteins in dyslipoproteine-mic patients. Circulation 1999;100(18 Suppl 1) [abstract: 1342].

38. Wetterau JR, Gregg RE, Harrity TW, et al. An MTP inhibitor that normalizes atherogenic lipoprotein levels in WHHL rabbits. Science 1999;282:751–4.

39. Farnier M, Stein E, Megnien S, et al. Efficacy and safety of implitapide, a micro-somal triglyceride transfer protein inhibitor in patients with primary hypercholes-terolemia. Abstract Book of the XIV International Symposium on Drugs Affecting Lipid Metabolism. New York, September 9–12, 2001. p. 4.

40. Available at: http://www.clinicaltrials.gov/ct/show/NCT00079859. Accessed June 10, 2008.

41. Cuchel M, Bloedon LT, Szapary PO, et al. Inhibition of microsomal triglyceride transfer protein in familial hypercholesterolemia. N Engl J Med 2007;356:148–56.

42. Available at: http://www.sec.gov/Archives/edgar/data/1338042/000119312 507123502/ds1a.htm. Aegerion Pharmaceuticals, Inc. Common Stock Registra-tion Statement. AMENDMENT NO. 3 to FORM S-1; May 25, 2007. United States Securities and Exchange Commission. Washington, DC. 20549. 2007. Ac-cessed July 12, 2014.

43. Samaha FF, McKenney J, Bloedon LT, et al. Inhibition of microsomal triglyceride transfer protein alone or with ezetimibe in patients with moderate hypercholes-terolemia. Nat Clin Pract Cardiovasc Med 2008;5:497–505.

44. Cuchel M, Meagher EA, du Toit Theron H, et al. Efficacy and safety of a micro-somal triglyceride transfer protein inhibitor in patients with homozygous familial hypercholesterolaemia: a single-arm, open-label, phase 3 study. Lancet 2013; 381:40–6.

45. Efficacy and safety of lomitapide in Japanese patients with HoFH on concurrent lipid-lowering therapy. Available at: http://clinicaltrials.gov/ct2/show/record/ NCT02173158?term=lomitapide&rank=8. Accessed July 12, 2014.

46. Stein EA, Raal FJ. Reduction of low density lipoprotein cholesterol by mono-clonal antibody inhibition of PCSK9. Annu Rev Med 2014;65:417–31.

47. Tall AR, Jiang X, Luo Y, et al. 1999 George Lyman Duff memorial lecture: lipid transfer proteins, HDL metabolism, and atherogenesis. Arterioscler Thromb Vasc Biol 2000;20:1185–8.

48. Clark RW, Sutfin TA, Ruggeri RB, et al. Raising high-density lipoprotein in hu-mans through inhibition of cholesteryl ester transfer protein: an initial multidose study of torcetrapib. Arterioscler Thromb Vasc Biol 2004;24:490–7.

49. de Grooth GJ, Kuivenhoven JA, Stalenhoef AF, et al. Efficacy and safety of a novel cholesteryl ester transfer protein inhibitor, JTT-705, in humans: a random-ized phase II dose-response study. Circulation 2002;105:2159–65.

50. Barter PJ, Caulfield M, Eriksson M, et al. Effects of torcetrapib in patients at high risk for coronary events. N Engl J Med 2007;357:2109–22.

51. Schwartz GG, Olsson AG, Abt M, et al. Effects of dalcetrapib in patients with a recent acute coronary syndrome. N Engl J Med 2012;367(22):2089–99.

52. Abifadel M, Varret M, Rabès JP, et al. Mutations in PCSK9 cause autosomal dominant hypercholesterolemia. Nat Genet 2003;34:154–6.

53. Maxwell KN, Breslow JL. Adenoviral-mediated expression of PCSK9 in mice re-sults in a low-density lipoprotein receptor knockout phenotype. Proc Natl Acad Sci U S A 2004;101:7100–5.

54. Maxwell KN, Fisher EA, Breslow JL. Overexpression of PCSK9 accelerates the degradation of the LDLR in a post–endoplasmic reticulum compartment. Proc Natl Acad Sci U S A 2005;102(6):2069–74.

55. Rashid S, Curtis DE, Garuti R, et al. Horton decreased plasma cholesterol and hypersensitivity to statins in mice lacking PCSK9. Proc Natl Acad Sci U S A 2005;102:5374–9.
56. Cohen JC, Boerwinkle E, Mosley TH Jr, et al. Sequence variations in PCSK9, low LDL, and protection against coronary heart disease. N Engl J Med 2006;354:1264–72.
57. Zhao Z, Tuakli-Wosornu Y, Lagace TA, et al. Molecular characterization of loss-of-function mutations in PCSK9 and identification of a compound heterozygote. Am J Hum Genet 2006;79(3):514–23.
58. Lagace TA, Curtis DE, Garuti R, et al. Secreted PCSK9 decreases the number of LDL receptors in hepatocytes and in livers of parabiotic mice. J Clin Invest 2006; 116:2995–3005.
59. Chan JC, Piper DE, Cao Q, et al. A proprotein convertase subtilisin/kexin type 9 neutralizing antibody reduces serum cholesterol in mice and nonhuman primates. Proc Natl Acad Sci U S A 2009;106:9820–5.
60. Berthold HK, Seidah NG, Benjannet S, et al. Evidence from a randomized trial that simvastatin, but not ezetimibe, upregulates circulating PCSK9 levels. PLoS One 2013;8(3):e60095. http://dx.doi.org/10.1371/journal.pone.0060095.
61. Stein EA, Mellis S, Yancopoulos GD, et al. Effect of a monoclonal antibody to PCSK9 on LDL cholesterol. N Engl J Med 2012;366:1108–83.
62. Dias CS, Shaywitz AJ, Wasserman SM, et al. Effects of AMG 145 on low-density lipoprotein cholesterol levels: results from 2 randomized, double-blind, placebo controlled, ascending-dose phase 1 studies in healthy volunteers and hypercholesterolemic subjects on statins. J Am Coll Cardiol 2012;60:1888–98.
63. Further Cardiovascular Outcomes Research With PCSK9 Inhibition in Subjects With Elevated Risk (FOURIER). Available at: http://clinicaltrials.gov/show/NCT01764633. Accessed July 12, 2014.
64. ODYSSEY outcomes: evaluation of cardiovascular outcomes after an acute coronary syndrome during treatment with Alirocumab SAR236553 (REGN727). Available at: http://clinicaltrials.gov/ct2/show/NCT01663402?term=odyssey&rank=6. Accessed July 12, 2014.
65. The evaluation of PF-04950615 (RN316), in reducing the occurrence of major cardiovascular events in high risk subjects (SPIRE-1). Available at: http://clinicaltrials.gov/ct2/show/NCT01975376?term=PF-04950615&rank=13. Accessed July 12, 2014.
66. McKenney JM, Koren MJ, Kereiakes DJ, et al. Safety and efficacy of a monoclonal antibody to proprotein convertase subtilisin/kexin type 9 serine protease, SAR236553/REGN727, in patients with primary hypercholesterolemia receiving ongoing stable atorvastatin therapy. J Am Coll Cardiol 2012;59:2344–53.
67. Roth EM, McKenney JM, Hanotin C, et al. Atorvastatin with or without an antibody to PCSK9 in primary hypercholesterolemia. N Engl J Med 2012;367:1891–900.
68. Stein EA, Gipe D, Bergeron J, et al. Effect of a monoclonal antibody to PCSK9, REGN727/SAR236553, to reduce low-density lipoprotein cholesterol in patients with heterozygous familial hypercholesterolaemia on stable statin dose with or without ezetimibe therapy: a phase 2 randomised controlled trial. Lancet 2012;380:29–36.
69. Giugliano RP, Desai NR, Kohli P, et al. Efficacy, safety, and tolerability of a monoclonal antibody to proprotein convertase subtilisin/kexin type 9 in combination with a statin in patients with hypercholesterolaemia (LAPLACE-TIMI 57): a randomised, placebo-controlled, dose-ranging, phase 2 study. Lancet 2012;380:2007–17.

70. Koren MJ, Scott R, Kim JB, et al. Efficacy, safety, and tolerability of a monoclonal antibody to proprotein convertase subtilisin/kexin type 9 as monotherapy in patients with hypercholesterolaemia (MENDEL): a randomised, double-blind, placebo-controlled, phase 2 study. Lancet 2012;380:1995–2006.

71. Raal F, Scott R, Somaratne R, et al. Low-density lipoprotein cholesterol-lowering effects of AMG 145, a monoclonal antibody to proprotein convertase subtilisin/kexin type 9 serine protease in patients with heterozygous familial hypercholesterolemia: the Reduction of LDL-C with PCSK9 Inhibition in Heterozygous Familial Hypercholesterolemia Disorder (RUTHERFORD) randomized trial. Circulation 2012;126:2408–17.

72. Sullivan D, Olsson AG, Scott R, et al. Effect of a monoclonal antibody to PCSK9 on low-density lipoprotein cholesterol levels in statin-intolerant patients: the GAUSS randomized trial. JAMA 2012;308:2497–506.

73. Blom DJ, Hala T, Bolognese M, et al, for the DESCARTES Investigators. A 52-week placebo-controlled trial of evolocumab in hyperlipidemia. N Engl J Med 2014;370:1809–19.

74. Koren MJ, Lundqvist P, Bolognese M, et al, MENDEL-2 Investigators. Anti-PCSK9 monotherapy for hypercholesterolemia: the MENDEL-2 randomized, controlled phase III clinical trial of evolocumab. J Am Coll Cardiol 2014; 63(23):2531–40.

75. Stroes E, Colquhoun D, Sullivan D, et al, GAUSS-2 Investigators. Anti-PCSK9 antibody effectively lowers cholesterol in patients with statin intolerance: the GAUSS-2 randomized, placebo-controlled phase 3 clinical trial of evolocumab. J Am Coll Cardiol 2014;63(23):2541–8.

76. Robinson JG, Nedergaard BS, Rogers WJ, et al, LAPLACE-2 Investigators. Effect of evolocumab or ezetimibe added to moderate- or high-intensity statin therapy on LDL-C lowering in patients with hypercholesterolemia: the LAPLACE-2 randomized clinical trial. JAMA 2014;311(18):1870–82.

77. Stein EA, Giugliano RP, Koren MJ, et al. Efficacy and safety of evolocumab (AMG 145), a fully human monoclonal antibody to PCSK9, in hyperlipidaemic patients on various background lipid therapies: pooled analysis of 1359 patients in 4 phase 2 trials. Eur Heart J 2014. http://dx.doi.org/10.1093/eurheartj/ehu085.

78. Raal FJ, Giugliano RP, Sabatine MS, et al. Reduction in lipoprotein (a) with the PCSK9 monoclonal antibody evolocumab (AMG 145): a pooled analysis of over 1300 patients in 4 phase 2 trials. J Am Coll Cardiol 2014;63:1278–88.

79. Stein EA, Honarpour N, Wasserman SM, et al. Effect of the proprotein convertase Subtilisin/Kexin 9 monoclonal antibody, AMG 145, in homozygous familial hypercholesterolemia. Circulation 2013;128:2113–20.

80. Raal FJ, Honarpour N, Blom DJ, et al. Inhibition of PCSK9 with evolocumab in homozygous familial hypercholesterolaemia (TESLA Part B): a randomised, double-blind, placebo-controlled trial. Lancet 2014.

81. The evaluation of PF-04950615 (RN316) in reducing the occurrence of major cardiovascular events in high risk subjects (SPIRE-2). Available at: http://clinicaltrials.gov/ct2/show/NCT01975389?term=PF-04950615&rank=14. Accessed July 12, 2014.

82. Graham MJ, Lemonidis KM, Whipple CP, et al. Antisense inhibition of proprotein convertase subtilisin/kexin type 9 reduces serum LDL in hyperlipidemic mice. J Lipid Res 2007;48:763–7.

83. ISIS Press Release. Bristol-Myers SQUIBB selects ISIS drug targeting PCSK9 as development candidate for prevention and treatment of cardiovascular disease. Carlsbad (CA): PRNewswire-FirstCall; 2008. Available at: http://ir.isispharm.

com/phoenix.zhtml?c=222170&p=irol-newsArticle&ID=1289499.   Accessed September 23, 2014.

84. Fitzgerald K, Frank-Kamenetsky M, Shulga-Morskaya S, et al. Effect of an RNA interference drug on the synthesis of proprotein convertase subtilisin/kexin type 9 (PCSK9) and the concentration of serum LDL cholesterol in healthy volunteers: a randomised, single-blind, placebo-controlled, phase 1 trial. Lancet 2014; 383(9911):60–8.

85. Thompson A, Di Angelantonio E, Sarwar N, et al. Association of cholesteryl ester transfer protein genotypes with CETP mass and activity, lipid levels, and coronary risk. JAMA 2008;299:2777–88.

86. Krishna R, Anderson MS, Bergman AJ, et al. Effect of the cholesteryl ester transfer protein inhibitor, anacetrapib, on lipoproteins in patients with dyslipidaemia and on 24-h ambulatory blood pressure in healthy individuals: two double-blind, randomised placebo-controlled phase I studies. Lancet 2007;370: 1907–14.

87. Nicholls SJ, Brewer HB, Kastelein JJ, et al. Effects of the CETP inhibitor evacetrapib administered as monotherapy or in combination with statins on HDL and LDL cholesterol: a randomized controlled trial. JAMA 2011;306(19):2099–109.

88. A study of evacetrapib in high-risk vascular disease (ACCELERATE). Available at: http://clinicaltrials.gov/show/NCT01687998. Accessed July 12, 2014.

89. REVEAL: randomized evaluation of the effects of anacetrapib through lipid-modification. Available at: http://clinicaltrials.gov/show/NCT01252953. Accessed July 15, 2014.

90. Bloomfield D, Carlson GL, Sapre A, et al. Efficacy and safety of the cholesteryl ester transfer protein inhibitor anacetrapib as monotherapy and coadministered with atorvastatin in dyslipidemic patients. Am Heart J 2009;157(2):352–60.

91. Cannon CP, Shah S, Dansky HM, et al. Safety of anacetrapib in patients with or at high risk for coronary heart disease. N Engl J Med 2010;363:2406–15.

92. Anacetrapib: Merck provides information about a different method to measure LDL cholesterol and progress on REVEAL study. Available at: http://www.mercknewsroom.com/press-release/research-and-developmentnews/merck-provides-update-cardiovascular-development-program. Accessed July 12, 2014.

93. FDA briefing document NDA 203858. Available at: http://www.fda.gov/downloads/AdvisoryCommittees/CommitteesMeetingMaterials/Drugs/Endocrinologicand MetabolicDrugsAdvisoryCommittee/UCM323841.pdf. Accessed July 16, 2014.

Index

Note: Page numbers of article titles are in **boldface** type.

Endocrinol Metab Clin N Am 43 (2014) 1035–1055
http://dx.doi.org/10.1016/S0889-8529(14)00088-7
0889-8529/14/$ – see front matter © 2014 Elsevier Inc. All rights reserved.

endo.theclinics.com

United States Postal Service

Statement of Ownership, Management, and Circulation
(All Periodicals Publications Except Requestor Publications)

1. Publication Title
Endocrinology and Metabolism Clinics of North America

2. Publication Number
0 0 0 - 2 7 5

3. Filing Date
9/14/14

4. Issue Frequency
Mar, Jun, Sep, Dec

5. Number of Issues Published Annually
4

6. Annual Subscription Price
$330.00

7. Complete Mailing Address of Known Office of Publication (Not printer) (Street, city, county, state, and ZIP+4®)
Elsevier Inc.
360 Park Avenue South
New York, NY 10010-1710

Contact Person
Stephen R. Bushing

Telephone (Include area code)
215-239-3688

8. Complete Mailing Address of Headquarters or General Business Office of Publisher (Not printer)
Elsevier Inc., 360 Park Avenue South, New York, NY 10010-1710

9. Full Names and Complete Mailing Addresses of Publisher, Editor, and Managing Editor (Do not leave blank)

Publisher (Name and complete mailing address)
Linda Belfus, Elsevier Inc., 1600 John F. Kennedy Blvd., Suite 1800, Philadelphia, PA 19103-2899

Editor (Name and complete mailing address)
Jessica McCool, Elsevier Inc., 1600 John F. Kennedy Blvd., Suite 1800, Philadelphia, PA 19103-2899

Managing Editor (Name and complete mailing address)
Adrianne Brigido, Elsevier Inc., 1600 John F. Kennedy Blvd., Suite 1800, Philadelphia, PA 19103-2899

10. Owner (Do not leave blank. If the publication is owned by a corporation, give the name and address of the corporation immediately followed by the names and addresses of all stockholders owning or holding 1 percent or more of the total amount of stock. If not owned by a corporation, give the names and addresses of the individual owners. If owned by a partnership or other unincorporated firm, give its name and address as well as those of each individual owner. If the publication is published by a nonprofit organization, give its name and address.)

Full Name	Complete Mailing Address
Wholly owned subsidiary of	1600 John F. Kennedy Blvd, Ste. 1800
Reed/Elsevier, US holdings	Philadelphia, PA 19103-2899

11. Known Bondholders, Mortgagees, and Other Security Holders Owning or Holding 1 Percent or More of Total Amount of Bonds, Mortgages, or Other Securities. If none, check box. ☑ None

Full Name	Complete Mailing Address
N/A	

12. Tax Status (For completion by nonprofit organizations authorized to mail at nonprofit rates) (Check one)
The purpose, function, and nonprofit status of this organization and the exempt status for federal income tax purposes:
☐ Has Not Changed During Preceding 12 Months
☐ Has Changed During Preceding 12 Months (Publisher must submit explanation of change with this statement)

PS Form 3526, August 2012 (Page 1 of 3 (Instructions Page 3)) PSN 7530-01-000-9931 PRIVACY NOTICE: See our Privacy policy in www.usps.com

---

13. Publication Title
Endocrinology and Metabolism Clinics of North America

14. Issue Date for Circulation Data Below
June 2014

15. Extent and Nature of Circulation

		Average No. Copies Each Issue During Preceding 12 Months	No. Copies of Single Issue Published Nearest to Filing Date
a. Total Number of Copies (Net press run)		955	901
b. Paid Circulation (By Mail and Outside the Mail)	(1) Mailed Outside-County Paid Subscriptions Stated on PS Form 3541. (Include paid distribution above nominal rate, advertiser's proof copies, and exchange copies)	465	418
	(2) Mailed In-County Paid Subscriptions Stated on PS Form 3541 (Include paid distribution above nominal rate, advertiser's proof copies, and exchange copies)		
	(3) Paid Distribution Outside the Mails Including Sales Through Dealers and Carriers, Street Vendors, Counter Sales, and Other Paid Distribution Outside USPS®	239	212
	(4) Paid Distribution by Other Classes Mailed Through the USPS (e.g. First-Class Mail®)		
c. Total Paid Distribution (Sum of 15b (1), (2), (3), and (4))	▶	704	630
d. Free or Nominal Rate Distribution (By Mail and Outside the Mail)	(1) Free or Nominal Rate Outside-County Copies Included on PS Form 3541	52	91
	(2) Free or Nominal Rate In-County Copies Included on PS Form 3541		
	(3) Free or Nominal Rate Copies Mailed at Other Classes Through the USPS (e.g. First-Class Mail)		
	(4) Free or Nominal Rate Distribution Outside the Mail (Carriers or other means)		
e. Total Free or Nominal Rate Distribution (Sum of 15d (1), (2), (3) and (4))	▶	52	91
f. Total Distribution (Sum of 15c and 15e)	▶	756	721
g. Copies not Distributed (See instructions to publishers #4 (page #3))	▶	199	180
h. Total (Sum of 15f and g)	▶	955	901
i. Percent Paid (15c divided by 15f times 100)	▶	93.12%	87.38%

16. Total circulation includes electronic copies. Report circulation on PS Form 3526-X worksheet.

17. Publication of Statement of Ownership
If the publication is a general publication, publication of this statement is required. Will be printed in the December 2014 issue of this publication.

18. Signature and Title of Editor, Publisher, Business Manager, or Owner

[signature]
Stephen R. Bushing – Inventory Distribution Coordinator

Date
September 14, 2014

I certify that all information furnished on this form is true and complete. I understand that anyone who furnishes false or misleading information on this form or who omits material or information requested on the form may be subject to criminal sanctions (including fines and imprisonment) and/or civil sanctions (including civil penalties).

PS Form 3526, August 2012 (Page 2 of 3)

Moving?

Make sure your subscription moves with you!

To notify us of your new address, find your **Clinics Account Number** (located on your mailing label above your name), and contact customer service at:

Email: journalscustomerservice-usa@elsevier.com

800-654-2452 (subscribers in the U.S. & Canada)
314-447-8871 (subscribers outside of the U.S. & Canada)

Fax number: 314-447-8029

Elsevier Health Sciences Division
Subscription Customer Service
3251 Riverport Lane
Maryland Heights, MO 63043

*To ensure uninterrupted delivery of your subscription, please notify us at least 4 weeks in advance of move.

Printed and bound by CPI Group (UK) Ltd, Croydon, CR0 4YY

03/10/2024

01040492-0019